TURN ON YOUR INNER LIGHT

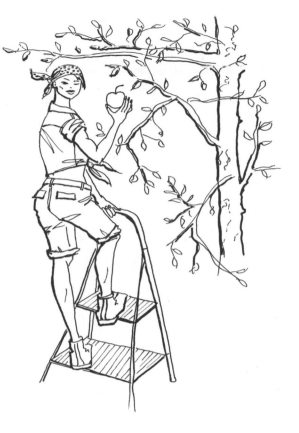

FITNESS FOR BODY MIND AND SOUL

DEBBIE EISENSTADT MANDEL

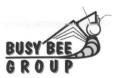

BUSY BEE GROUP

TURN ON YOUR INNER LIGHT
FITNESS FOR BODY, MIND AND SOUL
Debbie Eisenstadt Mandel

Published by:
Busy Bee Group
P.O. Box 327
Lawrence, NY 11559
busybeegroup.com

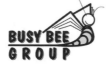

Fitness concepts and exercises: . . . . . . Frank Mikulka
Cover art and exercise illustrations: . . .Elena Markina
Cartoons: . . . . Brendan O'Connor
Book design: . . . . Steve Mandel
Cover design: . . . . .Dan Stoica

Publisher's Cataloging-in-Publication
(*Provided by Quality Books, Inc.*)

Mandel, Debbie Eisenstadt
Turn On Your Inner Light: Fitness for Body, Mind and Soul / Debbie Eisenstadt Mandel
p. cm
LCCN 2002092901
ISBN 0-9722166-9-3

1. Exercise. 2. Mind and Body. 3. Exercise—Miscellanea
4. Soul—Miscellanea. I. Title
RA781.M36 2003   613.7'1
QBI33-642

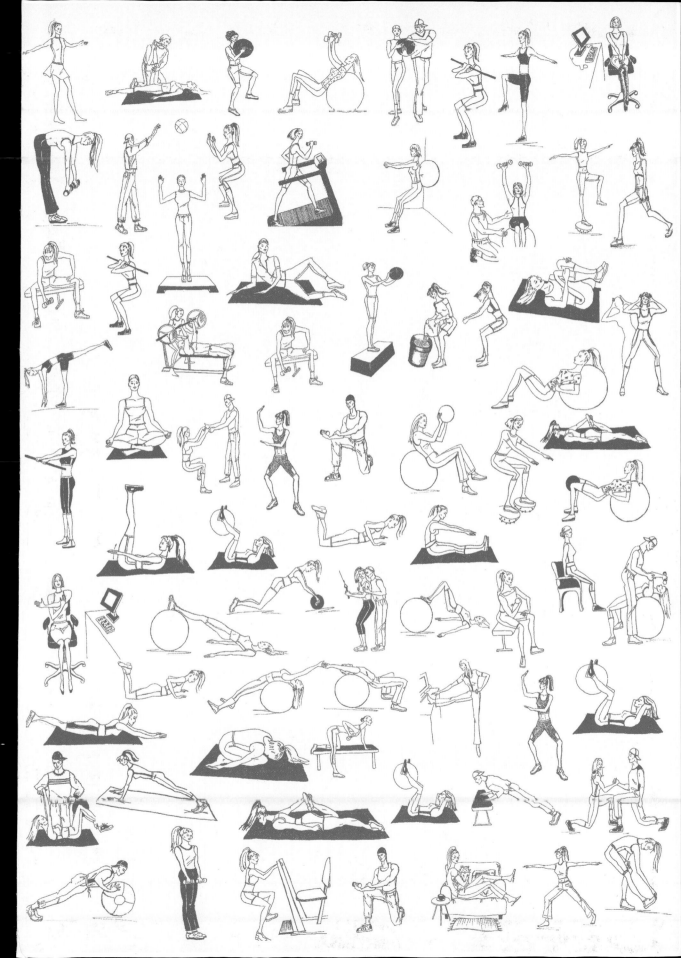

DEDICATION

TUNA GOLDMAN   SAMUEL ABRAHAM
EISENSTADT

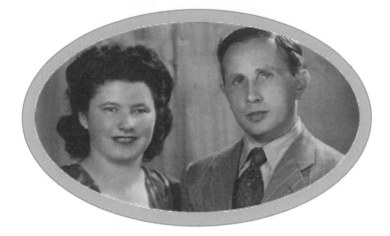

I dedicate this book to my parents, holocaust survivors, who reside both on earth and in heaven. They built a house furnished with unconditional love, joy and laughter. Growing up against the backdrop of the holocaust, I learned from an early age to appreciate the light and to value personal empowerment. My writing honors their goodness and creativity. Their spiritual legacy needs no testimony.

ACKNOWLEDGEMENTS

I thank my cousin, Esther Fingerhut Ettedgui, a hidden child during World War II and a self-made woman, for being a loving sister who gives me the most honest and intelligent "unsolicited" advice. Her energy, wit and intellect have been a driving force in my life.

I thank my children, Michael, David, Amanda and my daughter in law Lisi, for their love, humor and tolerance.

*A special heartfelt thank you to my husband, Steve, a mathematician with a wry sense of humor, who put up with my artistic temperament all these years (even before I became a writer) and for partnering the creative design and implementation of **Turn On Your Inner Light**. He anchors the flights of my fancy.*

Thank you: Mindy Frenkel, Abelardo Martinez, Dr. Stuart Rapapport, Dr. Abraham Abittan, Wendy Friend, Cheryl MacDavid, Eddie Ruane, Richard Brodsky, Kathy Mandel and Shifra Hanon for your help, intellectual support and optimism.

The following wonderfully talented people contributed to the synergy of the text:

Frank Mikulka, a trainer elite, martial artist and former Marine, is the fitness consultant for all the exercises. His Zen vision, expertise and motivating words created movements that mattered.

Elena Markina, a talented illustrator and painter, Brendan O'Connor, a creative cartoonist, and Dan Stoica, an imaginative cover designer.

A special thank you to Bernie S. Siegel, M.D. who inspired and then actually opened the door for me to bring this book into reality. Although I was not his patient, or someone he had previously worked with, he helped me a total stranger-- simply because I asked and he liked what I had to say. I have attended workshops by many writers and physicians, but the most authentically kind scientist I ever met is Bernie.

CONTENTS

FOREWORD

When we find ourselves in a dark room, we know what needs to be done. Go and find the switch that turns the light on. Some people prefer the dark because they are afraid to look at their reflection and others fear the dark because they do not realize they are capable of taking charcoal and turning it into a diamond. What is necessary in both cases? The pressure to change and the willingness to find guides and coaches who will teach you to change by becoming your trainer and re-parenting you. What you need to do is be willing to rehearse and practice to achieve a new and enlightened life, a rebirth. You can become a luminary, light the way and become a beacon for others. I am sure Debbie Mandel has had her share of troubles or she wouldn't be such a wise coach and trainer.

If you see your life as a time to train and learn, like going to school to be educated, this book can help make your life's experience a positive one. You will become a post-graduate student compared to others who are struggling to find themselves and their path. A big part of the problem relates to your willingness to achieve self-acceptance after growing up bombarded by the criticism of all the authorities in your life. However, constructive criticism can polish your mirror, as any good trainer, athlete or performer knows. So read and learn the way to enlightenment.

It will help if you are willing to deal with your past and your fears by becoming aware of the issues related to them. Your inner child needs to be loved and accepted no matter how others have treated you. Look at your baby pictures and move on. The past can be the motivating energy that moves you out of the darkness. Many personal health trainers had low self-esteem and self-images that led them to create a beautiful person out of an unloved child.

Your self image is the most important factor related to your health and well being. This is not about being perfect, but about being worth something and worth loving. You may have acted in an unwise manner, but you are loved and deserve to be cared for. Self-acceptance can be very difficult if parents, educators and clergy have bombarded you with feelings of guilt, shame and blame. Accept the criticism as guiding and instructing you and accept yourself as the worthy child of our Creator, which we all are.

Two things get us through tough times. They are love and laughter. You must start with self-love and the ability to become childlike in viewing the world. Then you will be able to laugh and survive. Love will be your building blocks and laughter the cement that holds them together. When you have those two factors, then the information in this book will be of value. If you do not have inspiration and enlightenment, there is no point in gathering information you will never use.

Find meaning in your life and you will choose a path that is not a dark tunnel, but a sunlit journey where there are no shadows because you are always facing the sun.

A poor man entered a dark cave one day to rest and when his eyes adjusted to the dark, he saw an enormous jewel reflecting the light. He reached out for it only to hear a frightening growl and see a large serpent guarding the jewel. He ran in fear and spent his life thinking how, if he had had the courage to pick up the jewel, his whole life would have been changed. When he was an old man, he decided to go back to the cave to see the jewel once again before he died. He entered the cave and there sat the jewel. As he moved towards it, he heard a little noise and looked into the darkness and saw a little lizard standing over the jewel. He picked up the jewel and took it home to his children, as a gift, to make their lives easier.

If you are ready to enter the cave, become a luminary and see that there is nothing to fear, read on. If not, go and find someone with a flashlight.

Peace,

Bernie S. Siegel, M.D.

PREFACE

Life is a series of training sessions. We train our minds, our muscles and our hearts. We train to win gracefully, to accept joy and we train to lose gracefully and accept sorrow. We train to give birth, but we do not train to be parents. We train to be productive for the first half of our lives, but we do not train for old age. We need to learn to fill in the gaps of living. Living is not synonymous with existence. It is about quality and exuberance, a renewed daily joy. Going through the motions with momentum means distraction, the avoidance of immersing our minds and bodies in the experience.

Turn on Your Inner Light is a self-help book providing spiritual guidance to release our brilliant light. Each one of us is born to shine. However, sometimes we suppress and are fearful of our individual power. This book offers a gentle and witty reminder to liberate our light when it is darkened by various life situations. In addition, the book presents fitness workouts to help our bodies connect with our spirits. When mind and body achieve balance, we become powerful beyond measure. Training teaches focus, discipline and feeling. We learn to become attuned to our bodies, control our movements, as we garner strength and energy. Ironically, the fatigue experienced at the end of a set, as muscles are literally torn down, creates greater strength and increases energy as muscle tissue almost immediately begins to repair and rebuild. Such opposition or dualities, the yin-yang of things, become inherent in training. This is the reason fitness experts like to work opposing muscles groups to strengthen a particular part of the body. Also, the mental and physical aspects of training combine to release a powerful energy: our inner light.

If we play a word association game with "train," we think of railroad, tunnels, tracks, roaring, derailment, and sex. Like a train we pass through dark tunnels and different land-scapes surprised at how quickly everything has passed by, or how quickly familiar landscapes have changed. Usually we visualize a training session in a fixed place, such as a gym. However, training can take place at home, or on vacation. And we can adjust to training in different landscapes because all training originates in the mind—the control center. Perception is everything. Like the little train that said, "I think I can, I think I can," if we say I think I can during workouts, then we can lift the weights, perform cardio-vascular activities, push ourselves to endure, control our movements, even do them gracefully. Movements are controlled from within. As we exercise our bodies, we exercise our minds increasing the blood flow to the brain, which sharpens our thinking and memory.

Endorphins are released making us feel excited, providing us with a sense of well-being, of renewed optimism. So if we don't have the luxury of a nearby gym during the course of our journey, we can always find creative substitutes such as, jump ropes, dyna bands, wrap around weights, free weights, even bottles, canned goods, balls, rocks, and the resistance of our own bodies.

Another word association for train is more widely known in literary circles, for a train is a literary symbol for sexual intercourse. A roaring train passing through a tunnel concretely demonstrates the male-female love connection. How appropriate to apply this image to training since it has been proven that training increases libido. When one looks good and feels attractive because his or her muscles are toned and the body is lean, then that person is less inhibited during sex and more open and receptive to one's lover. Too often, a person who feels unattractive about being naked is more concerned with covering up or hiding the body during sex than surrendering to the passionate moment. Also, aside from improving appearance, training increases blood flow to the sexual organs, raising testosterone levels in both males and females, which is responsible for heightened libido. All that is needed after a physical training session is to send an erotic message to the brain to combine blood flow with desire to experience sexual intimacy.

Training connotes learning how to live more intensely and with greater awareness under all conditions and situations. It suggests creativity, learning how to invent, to substitute and increase flexibility.

The purpose of this book is to instill mind/body workouts with a benevolent wit and a fresh eye for the unusual, or the unorthodox, to target specific life experiences like: romance, divorce, aging, sadness, failure, fear, addiction, conformity, talking too much and handling money. Original meditations reinforce each chapter's message. As in meditation, when one lifts weights, stretches, performs yoga postures or does cardio, he is both an observer and a participant. Of course, he is a participant because he is doing the actual work. However, it is not as obvious how he becomes an observer, which is equally as important, if not more important than the action or movement itself. On the most basic level one has to observe that he maintains proper form. On another level if one is really committed to the session, one maintains the focus of an observer to perform the one or two repetitions that recruit the greatest endurance from within, effecting the greatest changes in the body and ultimately the mind. As the body grows stronger, so does the mind and as the mind grows stronger, so does our ability to ward off illness.

As our bodies age, wrinkle, droop and sag, become mottled and gnarled, we do not realize that our minds are changing as well. Internal change is not superficial or as easily visible as the external. By teaching our bodies to lift, contract, straighten, and smooth out those extra, unwanted severe lines, our minds are also being taught to participate in this youth regenerating experience. The result of this mind/body connection is to set physical as well as spiritual goals to generate happiness. As the poet Dylan Thomas wrote, "Do not go gentle into that good night." No matter how old we are, we can still generate sparks, if not fireworks. Perception is all that matters. Feeling that our bodies can still do our bidding, and that our minds can suffuse our bodies with energy, inspiration and control, what stands in the way of realizing our endless possibilities?

What sets this mind/body/fitness book apart from the rest of its genre is that it provides a creative merger of spirituality and fitness. Targeted are people with specific social or health goals that are not often addressed. The ultimate goal is prevention not only treatment of disease or dis-ease. Skimming the table of contents will immediately evidence a broad spectrum of subjects such as training for: gardening, vulnerability, sensuality as well as, insomnia, technology, psychosomatic ailments and people who push our buttons. Training teaches one to live life connected both in body and spirit to experience the moment intensely. And when necessary, we can scale those insurmountable walls which come our way, one surefooted movement at a time; we even realize when to yield, to rest our bodies and redirect our movements to a different, friendlier, more open path that elicits our best abilities, rather than crush them as we beat our heads against a dense wall.

Training both the mind and the body provides a time and place to excel. Above all, the theme uniting the various chapters is--fun. Working out is fun. Our blood is pumping, our hearts are beating; our minds are clear; we are poetry in motion. We are in a heightened state of awareness, a concrete hour of accomplishment, time set aside to get in touch with our true inner child who has been hidden by life's many layers, or the daily multiple roles we juggle blocking his emergence. When we release this inner child, the world better watch out! We can then regain control of our lives, become our true selves, feel uninhibited by conformity and make ourselves vulnerable to emotional experiences. We stretch our contracted selves to powerfully grasp the golden ring. The process becomes more important than the end! And the process is fun!

Turn on Your Inner Light will help the reader shed many fears, including the fear of our own light; that we are too bright and that others will feel insecure next to us. When we let go of this basic fear, we let our true light shine. We inspire others to do the same.

When participating in a fitness program, many individuals choose to work with a personal trainer, an interesting title since it connotes the close relationship between client and trainer. Also, the title suggests that the training process strives for personal improvement, to cultivate and develop the total individual-- mind and body. The trainer contracts the client's world into sets of small personal goals. The client feels the trainer's positive energy, taps into it to reach deep within to do the extra repetition, go for the burn. When the client is ready to give up, fall down at the last push-up, his trainer reminds him to use the third eye located in the middle of the forehead to keep going without squirming until the sticking point is reached.

Some choose to work with a personal trainer for a short period of time to learn proper form and workout principles necessary to achieve the goals set for the body in terms of aerobic, anaerobic and stretching exercises. The goal shared between teacher and student seeks to make the student self-sufficient, in charge of his own body and muscular destiny.

However, many trainees have shared long, successful relationships with their aerobics instructors, yoga teachers and weight trainers who constantly move them, from one level to the next, helping them perform the seemingly insurmountable. Friendships, even life-long bonds, are formed; in these cases the lines blur between trainer and trainee. Sometimes in a humorous transference the trainer becomes the trainee and vice versa. During this session confidences are shared as well as anecdotes about the human condition. Training becomes a form of psychotherapy or the confessional between priest and parishioner. Mutual respect is exchanged as well as mutual well wishing, for their achievement becomes one. If the student looks good, then the teacher looks good! It's as simple and as complex as that.

A good trainer creates a symbiotic relationship, for one learns by teaching. However, a great trainer makes the client feel as though every repetition counts in a noncompetitive environment because everyone depends on it; as though the client were a human bridge where a whole platoon, women and children must cross to safety in order to avoid falling into the abyss; or a human ladder during a fire leading the family to safety. Training teaches one to be functional on the outside world, emotionally and physically, to think clearly during a stressful situation and to act with strength and conviction during emergencies.

When I first started training seven years ago with my first personal trainer who has since become a close friend, our relationship was one of opposition: She was muscular, sinewy, in fact, a strong thirty-five year-old woman who could lift weights and perform as well as, or even outperform men, and I a petite, soft woman with not a single toned muscle in her body. Thin calves and small arms led people to believe I needed protection, a helpless female. I could have worn a petticoat along with a hoop skirt, a bonnet and a parasol, for I looked the part of a fragile belle. Upon closer examination, as my trainer shook her head at the work cut out for her, with an "Oh, dear! Let's see what we can do here!" as confidences were exchanged and personalities emerged during the sessions, it became apparent that what we had was a case of dualities. Much was happening beneath the surface that the casual eye could not detect.

During my first session I, a woman of forty-three at the time, was put through my paces. She wanted to see at what point I would break. But I, a high impact aerobics queen, who could play singles tennis for three hours straight, would not surrender to this new, unfamiliar muscular challenge. At one point, my trainer leaned into me as I sat in the chest press machine, having soundlessly completed a grueling three sets, "You're not a screamer, are you?" I thought she couldn't possibly have said what I thought she said and meant it metaphorically like I thought she did. "What did you say?" I double-checked the question as I was feeling exhausted by the heavy weights. She repeated it verbatim. I looked into her mischievous brown eyes and I, certainly one to dissect every word, unabashedly and defiantly admitted, "No, I'm not!" We both understood one another and laughed loudly in abandon, girlishly. She realized I was not inhibited and judgmental, that she could tell me anything as I intuited the same about her at that very moment. When our eye beams intertwined at that point of mutual recognition, we decided we would be the best we could be for each other. I was the cerebral side, the cynic, the voice of reason. I believed only in the empirical and laughed at any hint of the mystical. She had never met a woman with as much inner strength and steeliness as me. How ironic to be captive in a petite, delicate, soft body! I often expressed that I would gladly give her some of my inner strength. And there she was my beautiful trainer. Olive skinned, long cascading black hair, a steely body housing a soft, fearful heart. During the course of four years there have been confidences exchanged, therapy sessions between us as we trained together both inside and outside of the gym and magically, opposing personality traits that have infiltrated each other's core.

My personal trainer, my female confidante, has taught me to feel, to allow myself to become more vulnerable to connect my mind with my body instead of being all mind. And in turn, she has become more reasonable, stronger on the inside, confronting her fears courageously and moving on instead of remaining paralyzed by them. She has connected her heart with her mind. In the beginning she was all talk of the spirit world, of previous lives, of feelings that cry out for validation. On the other hand, I laughed at her and called her a white witch; "I need proof!" I shouted. Together our journey has led to a transference of our better qualities. Now I am more muscular, substantial on the outside, but softer, more connected to my feelings on the inside, letting down walls constructed over the years; while she is now considerably stronger on the inside matching her exterior. During our past training sessions we have both learned balance. Even though we continue to differ, argue, fight, cry and laugh, we have trained not only our minds and our bodies, but also our tolerance for our differing perspectives. She has even got me saying; "We must have known each other in a previous life!" "Yes, you are an old soul," she says emotionally. "Who are you calling old?" I break up the emotional moment. We are still who we are. Training doesn't rearrange the molecules and create a new individual. Training makes one a more balanced, stronger individual alert to changes in the body as the mind tells the body what to do.

The chapters in this book offer spiritual guidance, exercises for the mind and body, quotes, witticisms, anecdotes, original meditations-- recipes for living. Improving the quality of life, heightening our senses and creating an open channel for happiness are the optimistic goals of this health guide. Also, the workouts are user friendly and have been created by a fitness professional, Frank Mikulka, with decades of experience. As in finding a workout partner, a friend, or a mate, the readiness is everything. The ultimate question: are you ready?

HOW TO USE THIS BOOK

Turn On Your Inner Light: Fitness for Body, Mind and Soul provides spiritual, physical and practical guidance for 29 common life situations. In each chapter you will find;

- An inspirational quote.
- Textual material presenting creative solutions for stressful situations.
- Mind/body prescriptions with hands-on concrete methods to achieve well being.
- An original meditation.
- Specific corresponding fitness sketches showing proper form along with clear and detailed easy to follow instructions.

The pages of *Turn On Your Inner Light* are meant to be flipped through regularly. The meditations will create serene interludes in the brain over the course of time. Each time you meditate, you will feel restored as though you have returned from a mini-vacation. The workouts are progressive ranging from beginner to the more advanced. As you perform the exercises, you will grow stronger, develop more endurance and feel more energetic. They will help you organize your day in a healthy way and provide you with physical affirmations to increase happiness. If you can't sleep and feel burned out, sad, angry, or have forgotten how to live in the moment, have fun, or be romantic, the various chapters will provide you with holistic "recipes" for living.

You can read through the chapters in any order you wish. You will enjoy reading the entire book even if you do not as yet identify with every life situation. Reading through these chapters will prepare and remind you of concepts that will empower you to live life in greater awareness and with more compassion. For example, even if you are not a senior citizen yet, you will be someday, or you have parents, or grandparents who wish to have their needs understood and met.

THE SUN WILL COME UP TOMORROW, BUT WHAT IF IT DOESN'T FOR YOU?

Certain people might need professional care such as that provided by a therapist or a physician to help them with more serious conditions. *Turn On Your Inner Light* does not presume to be a substitute for professional care. Use the tips, techniques and illustrations to stimulate self-awareness for greater vitality and happiness.

BEFORE
YOU EXERCISE

Before you begin any exercise program, consult your doctor. The author and fitness professional do not assume any responsibility for the exercises depicted in this book, particularly regarding individual performance, or personal debility. The reader performs these physical activities at his/her own risk. However, if you choose to follow the suggested workouts, then make sure to incorporate the following **consistently** in your routine.

- Maintain a balanced diet to fuel muscles and burn fat.
- Drink plenty of water to avoid dehydration and help flush out toxins.
- Do a five minute warm-up to help you find your focus and intensity, as well as to prevent injury.
- Maintain proper body alignment when executing an exercise; a mirror can help.
- When weight training, do not use momentum. Do each repetition slowly and carefully, imaging the mind-muscle connection.
- Hold abdominals in tightly to help support the back and create body stability.
- Don't hold your breath. Breathe rhythmically -- exhaling upon exertion.
- Always remember to stay in the moment. Focus by visualizing a specific muscle doing the work, connecting muscle and mind.
- Stop if you feel any pain or dizziness. Distinguish pain from "a burn" that is felt in the last few repetitions of weight training.
- Make sure to stretch after your workout to increase flexibility and prevent injury to muscles and connective tissue.
- Incorporate rest periods (a day or two) between workouts to let muscles recover and repair.
- Create a balanced program alternating between weight training and cardio components.
- Keep advancing in your workouts and change them periodically to stimulate your body and promote development. The body adapts to continued routines.
- Visualize an attractive, healthy and strong new you.
- Have fun.

CHAPTER 1

TRAINING TO BE CONSCIOUS

'Tis the mind that makes the body rich
Shakespeare

Stressful lifestyles prompt us to engage in the process of self-exploration. Scan the shelves in every bookstore, watch talk shows, or attend support groups, and you will observe others searching for greater meaning for spiritual answers to cope with fatigue, pessimism, anxiety and sadness. A question usually asked in some shape or form during workshops, "When you die, how would you introduce yourself to God or a higher power?" translates to: how do you define yourself? The answer provides the first step for connecting mind with body.

Traditionally, the conventional route to self-realization has been the therapist, the guide to the subconscious mind and the distant past. Nowadays tactile "psychologists" playing new age music while wafting various aromatic scents perform massage treatments using hot rocks, acupressure points, polarity and reflexology. Healing circles meet on beaches or in homes to meditate and join hands sharing positive energy to bolster the spirit, cultivating an eye for joy. Many hands-on-healers end a session by burning sage to cleanse the spirit. In other words, five individual senses are stimulated to make us aware of the sixth. However, let us not overlook the spiritual component of physical exercise as a means to self discovery and clear focus. Exercise helps us to feel alive, *to live in the moment* and the moment may be all that we have.

Being *conscious* is all about being mindful of what we do. When we feel fatigued at work, it is not work that is making us tired, but all the mental clutter that we bring to work. We think about elderly parents, our children's problems, a co-worker getting more attention from the boss, or the boss taking credit for our work. If we just did our work, we would not come home tired. We might even enjoy it!

WHERE TO ADD CONSCIOUSNESS IN OUR DAILY LIVES:

- **Nutrition** - We have to remember to eat! Many of us, frenetically juggling family and work, forget to eat. We eat on the run, quickly swallowing our food at fatty, salty, fast food places, barely conscious of the taste. We need to savor our food, conscious of its aroma and texture, chewing slowly. Also, we tend to get dehydrated, forgetting that we need to drink about eight glasses of water a day, depending on exertion and heat. We should try to eat a balanced diet of complex carbohydrates and proteins, cutting down on sugar and caffeine to avoid a rush as well as to properly and consistently fuel the body to stay alert and to prevent irritability.

- **Sleep** - If we don't get enough sleep, or have quality sleep, we feel depleted. When we dream at night, we sort out our day. If we are sleep deprived, we are not truly conscious during our day; we tend to get annoyed; we work and drive carelessly.

- **Weather** - Affects our bio-rhythms. In the winter when sunlight decreases, depression increases, Seasonal Affective Disorder. If we are aware of SAD, we know how to restore happiness with light.

- **Body signals** - Pain and fatigue signal us to be conscious of our thought patterns and lifestyles. Pain alerts us that something is wrong not only with our bodies, but with our minds. By understanding what emotional or thought driven issues make us sick and tired, we heal.

- **The subconscious** - Signals us in symbols through dreams, images and words. If we can decode its messages on a *conscious* level, we function more freely.

- **The good in our lives** - We tend to dwell on the negative, the small stain on the shirt, rather than the whole attractive garment. We need to appreciate the good in our lives. If we have a chronic illness, or have lost a job, we need *not label* ourselves by the negativity and become completely absorbed by it. "Hi, my name is Joe and I'm un-employed…" Or, the person who talks about his disease during the course of an entire dinner. We are so much more…

- **Living in the present** - Looking to the past and worrying or hoping about a future that might never happen drain us from living in the present. The present is a gift.

- **Love** - We need to see and be receptive to the love in our lives. Love expands our energy and sense of well-being.

- **Forgiveness** - Even when we are "right," we can re-interpret the scene with compassion and forgiveness. Being right and stressed is poor consolation.

- **Smiling** - Raises serotonin levels. Just turning up the corners of your mouth already accomplishes this. And when you smile, others want to be around you.

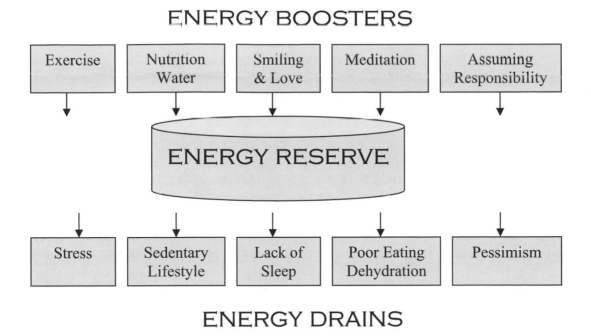

WHY DO WE WANT TO BE MORE CONSCIOUS?

We need to become aware of *energy boosters* and *energy drains*. We need to know what depletes us and costs us our vitality, our joy of living. For example, eating sugary products gives us a sugar rush, but then we crash and feel depleted soon after. On the other hand, eating a balanced diet sustains us throughout the day. If we know that we suffer from SAD, then we can raise the blinds, go outside in natural light, or even turn on bright fluorescent lights to feel happier and energized. Anger and pessimism are energy drains while optimism, compassion and appreciation are energy boosters. When we identify the boosters and drains of energy, we can change our perspective to increase empowerment.

Most importantly, we need to be conscious of stress in order to release its powerful energy drain and to quickly decompress. Because we are bombarded by four types of stress *simultaneously*: environmental, physical, internal and national, we need to know what they are in order to protect ourselves. Environmental stress consists of air and water pollution, radiation, food additives, pesticides, cleansers, chemicals, etc. Physical stress includes bacteria and viruses that visit or inhabit our bodies. Internal stress means unrealistic expectations, grief, and relationship woes. Our national vulnerability to terrorism causes us to live in anxiety and uncertainty. No wonder we feel overwhelmed and depleted! Because stress is enmeshed in our lives, we need the following process to restore balance.

COPE
CONSCIOUSNESS OBJECTIVITY PRACTICE ENERGY

FIVE SURE STEPS TO BE USED TO SHIFT FROM THE NEGATIVE ENERGY OF STRESS TO POSITIVE ENERGY

1. Identify the stressful situation and the accompanying feeling. Are you sad, angry, or anxious? Notice where the stress is lodged in your body. For example, does your neck, lower back, stomach, or head hurt?

2. Start to breathe consciously inhaling and exhaling to your own rhythm, sending your breath to the part of your body that feels stressed. Breathe consciously for about ten breaths. Also, it helps to say aloud or to yourself as you are breathing: "with each breath I am calming down, easing my heart." This replaces the old count to ten method. Your heart rate will slow down and you will start to relax just because you are bringing awareness to your breathing, a bodily function about which we are usually not conscious.

3. Visualize your stress. Give it shape, color and size. See it as a big picture, a mural.

4. Step back. You are standing too close to the big picture. Detach. Pretend it is your *friend's* problem. What would you advise a friend to do? We are adept at giving other people advice.

5. Reinterpret the picture. Shed the negativity of anger and resentment. Try to bring loving feelings into your consciousness: forgiveness, compassion and appreciation. See the positive side. Restore health and energy to mind and body.

Keep practicing to detach from the picture and introduce loving feelings in your interpretation. You might have to use **COPE** throughout the day. Soon the process will become automatic. *Note*: at the source of your stress lies your interpretation, which may have nothing to do with the reality of the actual situation. Two people might witness the same incident and see it differently.

The following is a personal example of the effectiveness of **COPE**: Recently, I leased my mother's apartment in her two family home as a summer rental. As soon as the new tenants moved into the apartment, the other, *permanent* tenant, a single woman with two cats, called me at eight thirty in the morning; she was filled with anger, barely able to speak: "Do you know that the new tenants parked their car so close to my side entryway that I had to shimmy through the neighbor's bushes where I tore my blazer coming home from my second job at midnight! How dangerous for me in the dark, a woman alone! Then I hear the machines going in the laundry room. I go down to the basement. What a mess! Clothes all over the floor and *she* puts *my* detergent away in the closet, while *she* puts *hers* out! *They* are inconsiderate, messy people who are taking over!"

Here was a need to practice **COPE** to defuse the situation. "Barbara, visualize your stress. What do you see?" "What do I see? Well, I see red!" "Where do you feel your stress? I feel it in my head. I have a terrible headache." "Barbara, breathe. Inhale and exhale. Breathe mindfully. Inhale and exhale." "What? I'm at work. Are you making fun of me?" "No, just bear with me. Please, inhale and exhale ten breaths." A few moments later, her voice settled down into a normal cadence. "Now, step back from the picture. Detach, pretend this happened to your friend. What advice would you give a friend?" I heard her smile-- it was audible, almost a giggle. She started to get it. "Now, let's reinterpret the picture. The temporary tenants are here because they had a fire that gutted their home. Husband, wife and two small children have been living like nomads for six months. Probably, they didn't realize that they had parked too close to your entryway. As to the laundry on the floor and the machines going full speed ahead at midnight, running after two small children all day and moving into a new apartment, perhaps this was the only time they could do the laundry. Why don't you speak to them about the situation and reach a compromise? Maybe they never lived in a two family home before?" "Thanks, Deb. I feel so much better. I cried myself to sleep last night. I couldn't concentrate on my work this morning. When you put it this way, they weren't doing it to spite me, they just didn't realize. I'll knock on their door tonight and introduce myself and ask them to park lower down the driveway and to be a little neater in the laundry room since I use it too. Hey, I better get back to work. Good talking to you."

COPE worked. Barbara could now be mindful of her work instead of being drained by anger. She became conscious that there was another side to the story and realized about what she was truly angry. She felt that she had seniority and they were taking over, pushing her out. Instead, she became compassionate about their hardships and forgave them. As a result, she felt calmer and ready to be productive.

Another method for de-stressing when we feel generalized anxiety, agitation, or depression is exercise. When we exercise, although it appears that we expend energy, ironically, we boost our energy levels and clarify our thinking by bringing oxygen to the brain. Also, we become conscious of the mind/body connection. We forego the negative issue for awhile. Often when we begin exercising, we feel fatigued; however, after about ten minutes of exertion, our endorphins kick in and we feel alive and happier.

CONSCIOUS EXERCISE VS. UNCONSCIOUS EXERCISE:

Unconscious exercise means not actively thinking. For example, you could be taking a step class and following the instructor's moves, mirroring those moves without thinking about the muscles you are using, or feeling each move. Perhaps you are weight training and talking up a storm during your workout, inadvertently forgetting to breathe, just taking shallow breaths, or using momentum. Obviously, if you can talk while weight training, you are not conscious of the muscles you are working and will not get the full benefit of the exercise. When you take shallow breaths, your body tenses up as it is not getting a complete flow of oxygen. When you engage your breath fully and deeply from the abdomen, you release tension as well as visualize the contracting muscle where you are sending oxygen. Conscious exercise brings an awareness of the body in every movement, tight abdominals, controlled quadriceps lifts, or hamstring curls. It is not about bouncy movements or momentum.

Many of us have become *unconscious worker-outers* whether in aerobics class or during a weight training session. The instructor or the personal trainer moves us through his choreography, his script and we follow without engaging our minds. Recently, I watched amusedly as a woman on all fours performed hydrants, side leg lifts in rapid succession, while speaking on a cell phone. One of the trainers who happened to pass by corrected her spinal alignment as she continued to talk animatedly on the phone, not even noticing him. The next day I observed another woman running sprints on the tennis court while speaking breathlessly on a cell phone.

What kind of person follows an unconscious workout? Someone unable to make choices, running away from life's challenges. An unhappy person is more likely to say, "Tell me what to do. I don't want to think." You can always spot an unconscious exerciser in a gym because that person uses momentum, fast bouncy movements as a distraction from thought. Mind and body are disjointed. An unconscious exerciser usually takes many aerobic classes, but never stays for the cool down period, instead runs to the next workout, the treadmill, or climbs a stair master immediately after class; the body does not feel the exercise, for the mind does not perceive it. Ironically, the body never changes for the better. Quite the contrary, muscles are burned from too much cardio and the body tends to look more flaccid!

Metaphorically, unconscious movements suggest experiencing life unconsciously, unaware of feelings, both painful and joyous. The mind is denied the information

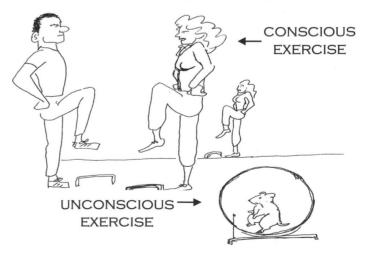

CONSCIOUS EXERCISE

UNCONSCIOUS EXERCISE

the body signals while the body does not receive the integrated evaluation and perception the mind transmits. How many of us eat popcorn at the movies without even realizing how much we are eating, or if we are hungry?

The solution: surrender to the experience, dig deeper into the self and think about the muscle group that is being worked. If you have two eight-pound weights in your hands and are doing biceps curls, you need to image the full extension as your arm unfurls on its way down like the taut ropes of a sail releasing tension. Then visualize the muscle tensing up from the biceps, not the hand or wrist, as the weight is driven upwards by the muscle. Each repetition should be performed as though it is the only one you are doing. Through this graphic, methodical visualization complete awareness can be achieved. The mind alertly pays attention to what the muscle is doing. And the muscle obeys the mind with proper form. When you visit a gym, notice the people who pay strict attention to form, how good their muscles look because their minds are focused on what their bodies are doing, as opposed to those who use rapid movements, relying on momentum to get them through their repetitions.

Once conscious movement becomes your goal in aerobics class or during strength training, life's experiences will take on a sharper, more intense imprint. Your workouts transfer to daily life. Denial, distractions and numbness exit from the unconscious mind to put the world into clearer focus, enabling the conscious person to exercise control and assume responsibility. Goals become clearer and commitments can be honored. Becoming conscious means stripping away the nonessentials to get to the essentials. We awaken to the joys of life's possibilities by living in the present.

When we synchronize thoughts with movements, the mind grows sharper, intuition heightens and happiness ensues. Whoever believed ignorance was bliss?

MIND/BODY PRESCRIPTIONS:

- ◆ Stir your coffee *backwards* to create awareness in routine activity.
- ◆ Take a *different* route to work to be conscious of the trip instead of driving on auto-pilot.
- ◆ Write an answer to the question: Where in your daily life would you like to be more conscious? Note that writing makes it come true.
- ◆ Hike on a natural terrain where you will have to memorize landmarks; create markers in your mind to find your way back.
- ◆ Make a list of things to appreciate. Also, make a list of things you used to appreciate, but have adapted to.

MEDITATION:

In the beginning many of us find it difficult to meditate, to concentrate on one image or phrase. Instead we review daily shopping lists, or compose to-do lists while our eyes are closed and our bodies are relaxed. We distract ourselves by life's clutter, to avoid thinking about the truth of our identity and the direction we are going. The reason for all this mental hustle and bustle is that we judge our thoughts. Instead if we could observe our thoughts float by, like leaves floating downstream, without any guilt or shame, we could achieve harmonious mind/body integration. This meditation will help the mind harness a focal point by imaging the body.

Sit up with dignity. Do not lie down, for you will be too relaxed and posture becomes important in meditation. Your spine should be erect to allow your energy to flow freely. Place the palms of your hands face down on your thighs to be in touch with your "inner knowing." Begin breathing deeply, inhaling from your nose and exhaling rhythmically from your nose. (If that is too difficult in the beginning, exhale from your mouth). Bring your attention to each distinct body part, tensing and releasing it. Begin with the head, the eyes, the mouth, the jaw; then move down to the neck, back, chest, arms, stomach, pelvis, legs and feet, one at a time. Notice after tensing each body part, your body begins to feel heavy, sinking into the floor, as your mind begins to open up. Now bring your focus to your third eye located in the space between your eyebrows. This is the center of your knowing. Visualize your clothes peeling away to reveal your skin. Allow your skin to dissolve to reveal your muscles. Feel your muscles melting until all that remains is your structure. Know that by stripping away, you are reaching your skeletal frame. Be conscious of your essential being. Within the apertures of your bones a golden light is revealed. This is your inner core. Be with your own golden light for a moment. Feel its glow. You can ask it anything that is on your mind right now. You will receive an answer, or what seems like nothing at all. It may be a word, an image, a color or a sound. It may appear now or come to you later in the day or in a dream. Wait a moment for the answer. Be receptive. Now let your muscles reattach to your skeleton. Let your skin smooth over each muscle. Your clothes reappear to cover your skin. With your eyes still closed, rub both of your hands together a few times as though they were two sticks about to light a campfire. Place both hands over your eyes. Feel your warm loving energy. Carry the consciousness of your essential being into your daily life.

EXERCISES TO CONSCIOUSLY PARTICIPATE: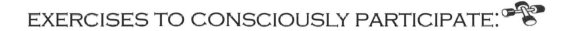

OBJECTIVE: TO BE IN THE MOMENT

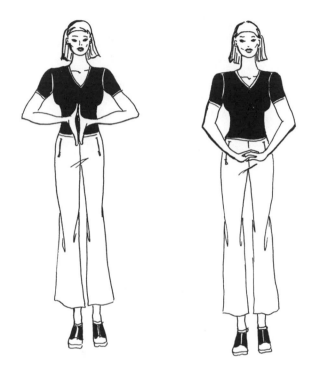

BREATHING

*Practice conscious breathing. Inhale and exhale through the nose. Inhale to a count of two; exhale to a count of four. Breathe deeply from the diaphragm. Feel your belly soften with the rise and fall of each breath. Do a series of 10. **Hint**: it helps to visualize your breath as a fog that you inhale with the in-breath and exhale with the out-breath.*

CONSCIOUS WALK *(Not Shown)*

Take a walk with a friend or group of friends around a track or in a prescribed area in your neighborhood where you have measured the distance. Set aside a specific time and commit to your friends to honor time and place. You will find that you and your group reinforce each other in this goal-oriented workout. After four to six weeks, set new goals. Walk at a faster pace, or for a longer distance. Eventually you might even consider alternating jogging with walking. The important point is to set a goal that the entire group strives to reach. This brings a new level of awareness to your workout.

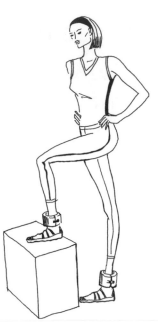

STEP UPS

Step up and down a foot-high box or bench for a set of 10 repetitions for each leg. Then strap on ankle weights 3-5 lbs on each leg. Do not look down, but keep your eyes straight ahead for good alignment. If you are not conscious of every movement, you might fall. A good idea is to have a partner stand next to you when you first practice this exercise. Do 3 sets of 8 repetitions with ankle weights.

SIDE LATERALS

Hold a 3 lb weight in each hand with your palms turned toward your body hands at your side in the starting position. Extend both arms in a side lateral raise. Point the head of the dumbbell downward with your pinkie pointed up as though you were pouring water. Make sure you lift the weights up and out to the sides so that they are slightly higher than shoulder level. Do not hyperextend. Do not swing the weights! Notice how your body is feeling. Close your eyes for the last 3 repetitions. Think of only your bones lifting the weight, not your muscles. Feel the bare essentials. Do a set of 8-10. Advance to 3 sets of 12 repetitions. Then when that feels easy, use 5 lb weights. In your last set after 6 repetitions, hold for 10 seconds in an iron cross position to break momentum. Then complete the set.

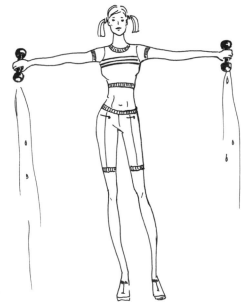

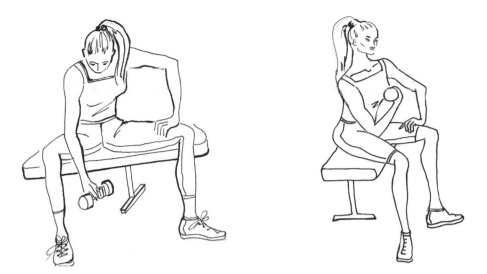

CONCENTRATION CURLS

*Do a concentration curl (biceps curl) that is driven purely from the biceps muscle and then returns to full extension. Do not recruit your wrist in the movement. Sit on a bench, coffee table, or low chair with your legs apart. Holding a dumbbell in your right hand, lean forward and position your arm, so that your elbow is pressed against your right inner thigh. With your palm facing up, curl the weight straight up. Go from full hang to an intense contraction felt in the biceps. Complete all the repetitions on your right side and switch to the left. Begin with 3 sets of 8 repetitions using a 5 lb weight. Gradually increase to 3 sets of 15 repetitions going up in weight, 8, 10 and then 12 lbs as the movements become easy. In the last set hold the weight midway for 10 seconds to break momentum. Then complete your set, making sure to return to full extension—do not cheat. **Hint**: As the workout gets harder, recruit your abdominals: hold them in tightly.*

THE SWAN

The Swan position increases strength, balance and endurance: Extend your arms horizontally and holding your abdominals in tightly, lift your knee up and hold for 5 seconds. Then alternate to the other knee. If you close your eyes, you can visualize your bones lifting. Do 8 on each side. As you advance increase the number of seconds you hold your knee up—20 seconds and do 3 sets.

CHAPTER 2

TRAINING FOR THE I DON'T HAVE THE TIME AND I HATE TO EXERCISE PERSON

There's a time for some things, and
A time for all things; a time for great
Things, and a time for small things
Miguel De Cervantes

Excuses grow more inventive and entrenched. "Oh, the reason you exercise so much is because you like it. But me, I hate exercising. I'm too tired; besides I always feel sore afterwards." "I'm too busy. I work all day and when I come home at night, I need to unwind." "I have small children; I'm too busy. I have no time for me." "I know exercise is important and that it's good for me; I just can't get motivated. I have no energy. I'd rather diet." However, for all the time it took to create these excuses, you could have been exercising!

Nowadays everyone is on a high stress alert. Our lives have become dramatic flourishes rivaled only by Shakespearean tragedies. We rush through daily existence from one activity to the next, juggling a full-time job with extended family and household responsibilities. Of course, we feel depleted and jittery. As a result, we smoke, or drink more caffeine to pump ourselves up. Then in keeping with our frenetic lifestyles, we eat fast foods high in fat, carbohydrates and sodium, quickly. We hardly sense the food hitting our stomachs, so we eat more to fill up on comfort food. Let us not forget chocolate, which is high on the comfort food list. As a result, we put on a few extra pounds. We grow disappointed with our appearance, feeling unhappy and start to compose a wish list, if only I could wear a smaller size, or lose ten pounds.

Why don't we exercise to make a change? At this point, perhaps, we fear that we will fail to lose the weight. After all, if we don't try, we can't fail. Some of us try to diet, denying ourselves pleasure, in order to look better. We work the whole day eating just a salad, or drinking a diet shake as we drive around from appointment to appointment, hungry. However, the body doesn't stay in a fasting mode for long; we return to our old eating habits with a vengeance, putting on even more weight than we lost.

The key to changing old patterns is to reset those rigid schedules. Sometimes you find yourself locked into a routine that needs to be reevaluated. Ask yourself what activities you

**GET IN SOME EXERCISE BY PARKING THE CAR
FURTHER AWAY FROM YOUR DESTINATION**

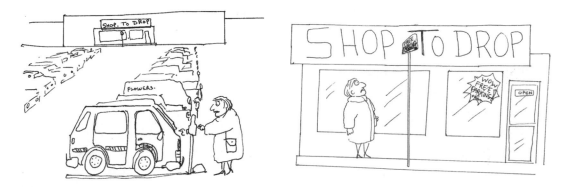

can delete from your program. If that doesn't work, then what if you woke up thirty minutes or an hour earlier every morning to exercise while everyone was still asleep in the house? You would have time for yourself to do something loving and positive. The flip side of this option is to exercise when everyone has gone to bed; however, since exercise is stimulating, you might not be able to fall asleep. The morning is best. A workout will inject you with energy and kick in those endorphins. If you workout before breakfast, perhaps drinking only a glass of orange juice, you will burn more stored fat.

Ironically, when you become too busy, things appear to fall apart in your personal life, going from bad to worse, because you grow distracted by the chaos. That is precisely when you have to release the old patterns and open yourself up to the changes that are occurring around you. The chaos bombarding your life is sending you signals from the universe. Slow down

THIS STRATEGY OCCASIONALLY BACKFIRES

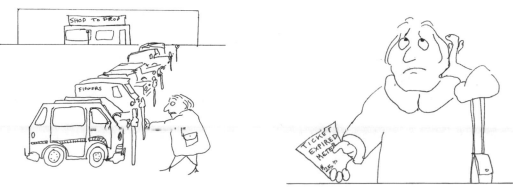

and contemplate what you need to learn about yourself in order to achieve more serenity.

Shedding your old skin to reveal the new layer does not usually happen quickly as it tends to be a lifelong process along with the fact that we have many layers to shed. You have to patiently commit to a new, healthier and benevolent lifestyle. Therefore when you want to shed those unwanted pounds to reveal your true self, the self you want to be, you need to involve your mind, visualizing who you are in a positive light. See yourself as beautiful and lovable within a realistic context. If you see yourself as not wanting to be fat, your brain focuses on the word fat, ignoring the word, "not." That is why many people continue to be heavier than they would like to be, unable to lose or maintain weight loss. However, if you see yourself as thin and gorgeous, then your brain will help the body fulfill that vision. Once your mind is clear about the vision, you need to create time and space as stepping stones for your physical and mental well being.

For instance, if you claim that you can't exercise for sixty minutes, or thirty minutes at a given time, perhaps you could start with ten minutes. What's ten minutes? Surely everyone can find ten minutes! You could even exercise for ten minutes twice a day and witness the gradual changes that occur in your body. Soon you will find another ten minutes until perhaps you have found four ten-minute periods during the day. Researchers feel that four short bursts of exercise can trigger as much, or even more weight loss than forty minutes straight! Invest in a treadmill or exercise bike for your home. The equipment is right there within reach; you don't have to waste time traveling to a gym. If you are ashamed of your appearance because of the extra weight you have put on and working out in public next to slim and trim bodies is putting salt on your wounded ego, then get into shape in the privacy of your home. Buy an exercise video appropriate for your level and participate with the members of the TV class.

When you have to drive to do various errands, don't park your car right next to your destination. Park your car a few blocks away and walk. Lifting and carrying packages to your car is a form of weight training. When you are in a shopping mall or office building, walk up the stairs, instead of using the elevator. You don't need a stair climber to find stairs to climb.

However, if you do join a gym, get a personal trainer to motivate you to do an intelligent workout, two to three times a week for a set time. A trainer will also design a personal program to be followed for the rest of the week. Immediately, you will feel better about the changes you have decided to make. Just scheduling that first appointment gives you a sense of control. Note: choose a personal trainer who is charismatic and has sex appeal. That will ensure that you work hard to please!

Interestingly enough, the more you exercise regularly, the more energy and strength you will have both mentally and physically to tackle life's struggles. Many of the time consuming or mentally consuming activities will appear trivial and unnecessary in your eyes, helping you to reevaluate the clutter and effectively creating more time for yourself. *Because anyone who cannot find even ten minutes for the self, is lost in the turmoil of existence.* And anyone who hates to exercise knowing its health promoting benefits, does not like the self very much.

Exercise changes the way the body processes food, making it easier for food to be burned as fuel rather than retained as fat. And when you lose pounds of fat, replacing the fat with muscle, you burn more calories even while you rest.

Exercise can prevent certain ailments like hypertension, late onset diabetes, and cardio-vascular disease, or at least delay their onset as well as help considerably in their management. An ounce of prevention is worth pounds and pounds of cure! While scientific advances have created medications to control blood pressure, cholesterol and glucose levels, unfortunately there are no cures for these conditions. Make self-care a priority through diet and exercise.

What is important for the harried, the distracted, I don't have time for myself person, is to begin to set aside a few moments every day. Make healthy living a priority. All your other activities depend on your health. Once you get sick with diabetes, or heart disease, it will create havoc in your schedule anyway! Exercise will actually help you organize your day differently—because it compels you to think about your health every day. Because a workout is hard work, you start to pay more attention to what you put into your mouth. After sweating for an hour to burn a few hundred calories, you are less likely to devour a candy bar. However, you must be ready. First, image the time and space in your mind. Visualize doing a workout, feeling stronger and looking better. Then do it in actuality, just as you imagined. This process needs a mind/body commitment to fully grow into a new healthier lifestyle. When beneficial physical changes take place in the body because of exercise, the mindset is changing along with the body to stimulate further development as well as to maintain this new lifestyle. The process becomes empowering because you have taken charge of your schedule and your life. You have exercised control!

MIND/BODY PRESCRIPTIONS:

- ♦ When you feel inundated with chores, slowly breathe; inhale and exhale. Close your eyes to focus inward as you feel your breath circulating throughout your body.
- ♦ Eat a balanced meal sitting down. When you eat right, you are giving yourself a message that you are important and that everything else can wait for you.
- ♦ Eat regularly; don't skip meals.
- ♦ Clean out your closets to clean out and organize the mental clutter. Rearranging your clothes and storage items based on usefulness, helps you to prioritize.

MEDITATION:

Lie down. Close your eyes. Inhale and exhale. Become one with your surroundings. Begin absorbing all the sounds and noises in the background. Go into your body and scan it for any aches or pains. Notice how you are feeling physically-- specifically. Accept it and move on. Be aware of how you feel emotionally. Are you sad, anxious, or worried? Label your emotion and let it go. Now begin to notice your breath. Sense the rise and fall of your abdomen. As you inhale, feel your chest and diaphragm expand filling your entire abdominal cavity with air. Pause and as you exhale, notice how your body releases tension. There is a natural pause between your breaths. Bring your attention to that moment. Experience your breath slowing down. Feel the health giving oxygen suffuse your entire being with every breath. Allow all the toxins to leave with every exhalation. As you inhale, your cells fill with energy. Experience this power surge. Isn't it wonderful to feel alive and restored? Gradually, open your eyes. Now that you have consciously experienced this energy, you know that all else depends on it. The next time you feel harried and stressed, restore yourself with this meditation. And if you don't have the time to meditate, simply become conscious of your breath and in so doing, you will naturally slow down.

EXERCISES FOR THE HATE TO EXERCISE PERSON:

OBJECTIVE: TO FIND THE TIME TO EXERCISE FOR THE RIGHT REASONS - HEALTH AND FITNESS

- *Listen to music with a rhythm that inspires you to move. Let your body dance to the rhythm. You can do this in a car when you are stuck in traffic. Move your shoulders, rib cage, waist and arms.*
- *Park your car a few blocks from your destination. Walk to wherever you have to go.*
- *Use the stairs at home, in department stores, or at work, instead of the elevator or escalator.*
- *Fantasize a positive vision of what you want to look like. Honor it and do something to make it come true: Conceive, believe, achieve.*

EXERCISES WHILE YOU WAIT IN LINE

*While waiting on the checkout line at the super-market, don't feel impatient; instead use the time to do the following: Kegels, contracting the urinary tract muscles and releasing, tightening the glutes and releasing, and holding in those abdominals. If you are more brazen, read a magazine to appear nonchalant as you lift a pointed straight leg a few inches off the ground and lower. Switch legs. If you are shy, do calf raises. Please see chapter 27, **Training in the Garden**.*

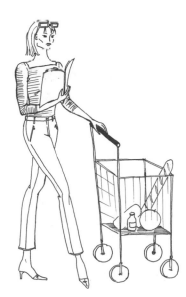

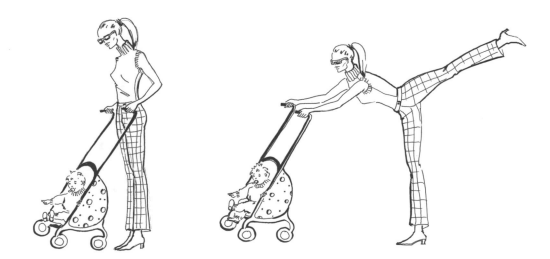

LEG EXTENSIONS WITH THE BABY IN A STROLLER

When pushing the stroller to air out the baby, you can intensify the exercise by extending your leg behind you as you tighten hamstrings and glutes and then lower almost touching the ground. Repeat on the other side. Do as many as you feel comfortable performing in public.

SIDE LEG LIFTS

Waiting? Use the time to do side leg lifts. Hold on to a cabinet, or television with one arm, and lift your straight leg to the side, a few inches off the floor. Return to touch your other leg, but do not touch the floor. Visualize that there is a weight on your calf as you lift and lower slowly and methodically. Switch sides. Do these until you are called.

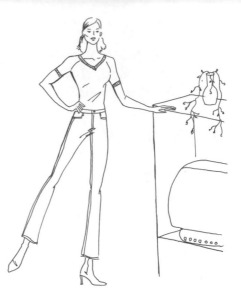

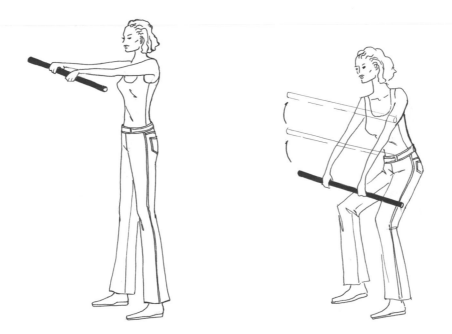

SQUAT WITH A BAR TO TARGET GLUTES AND SHOULDERS

*Try to maximize an exercise by doing 2 things at once. For example, squat with a bar extended in front of you in an overhand grip shoulder height. Lower the bar in synchrony every time you rise and lift the bar every time you squat. Do 8 repetitions. Then hold your squat position and lift the bar into 3 different raised positions. The uppermost position is level with your shoulders. Lower the bar down to your thighs from shoulder height as you stand straight. Do a set of 8 repetitions. For a detailed squat, please see chapter 3, **Training to Love Yourself**.*

TIPS TO SAVE TIME ON THE TRAINING FLOOR
TO GET IN AND OUT OF THE GYM QUICKLY
WITHOUT COMPROMISING INTENSITY

- *No socializing between sets.*
- *Start with a 5 minute meditation to help you focus.*
- *Work from larger to smaller muscle groups. Large muscle groups include: chest, back and legs. Small muscle groups include: triceps, biceps, shoulders and calves.*
- *Superset exercise pairs; for example, go from push-ups to pull-ups. When you finish a set of push-ups, immediately follow with pull-ups. No need to rest as these are opposing muscle groups.*
- *Do superset pairs for both lower and upper body. For example, do leg extensions for quadriceps immediately followed by hamstring curls. Another example is biceps curls followed by triceps extensions.*
- *Your breathing should be controlled and rhythmic during execution of exercise to make your body efficient upon exertion.*
- *Stretch at your convenience.*

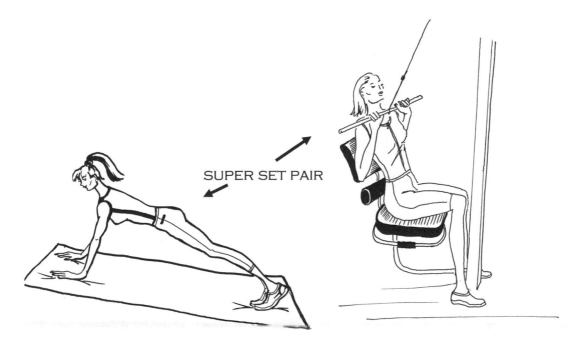

SUPER SET PAIR

CHAPTER 3

TRAINING TO LOVE YOURSELF

How do I love thee? Let me count the ways
Elizabeth Barrett Browning

Human beings are born complete and beautiful. The Bible tells us that we are created in God's image. As infants and children, we do not feel defective in any way. Then the people we encounter in our lives become our looking glass. We internalize their reflections as they communicate the beautiful things as well as the flaws they see. Because most of us want to conform to the aesthetic norm, which changes throughout the decades anyway, we become displeased with our outward appearance. We try to reshape ourselves, if we can, to suit these social pressures. Since many of us can't, we begin to dislike ourselves. Advertising agencies and the fashion industry point out ideals, not reality. Twenty five-year olds are photographed with anti-wrinkle creams. Svelte bodies model clothes for sizes 14 and up. We begin to feel that we don't measure up. As we internalize unrealistic expectations, we feel inferior and unattractive.

Meanwhile our daughters observe us. Young girls internalize their mothers' self-absorption with appearance. Daughters flinch at the criticism. "Are you sure you want to eat this ice-cream, dear?" A seven-year old pushes the plate away. "Don't you think those pants accentuate your stomach?" A teenager, who didn't think so before, does now. And even if we don't criticize our daughter's appearance, but take diet pills and skip meals, remember a little girl is watching us…

Animals have it a lot easier because they do not have to buy clothes. They don't look at their thighs and say they are too big. They don't look at their breasts and say they are too little. How many people, particularly women, would ever claim to be satisfied with their looks? Plastic surgery is thriving: redesigning noses and chins, lifting eyelids, faces and necks. Liposuction is sucking out fat deposits and reshaping bodies. Breasts are augmented not once, but even multiple times to keep up with the competition. "Mirror, mirror on the wall, who is the fairest of them all?" "You are" will not be the answer for very long.

Recently, I saw a woman staring at herself in the mirror in the gym. Every time she passed by a mirror she felt compelled to look at herself. She had undergone all the aforementioned surgical procedures by age 45. I realized that the reason she stared at herself in the mirror constantly, was that she didn't recognize who she was anymore!

Both men and women are susceptible to vanity, and a healthy amount of narcissism keeps us well groomed and looking the best that we can. Therein lies the difference between being obsessed with our looks and maximizing them. The age-old proverb about true beauty emanating from within is hard to believe in a youth-oriented society. Women feel especially vulnerable as they measure their personal attractiveness in a world of externals. They are competing for the attention of men who can be easily distracted by younger, sexier, more beautiful bodies that are constantly emerging. To be fair about it, women are seeking men who look, handsome, rugged and well-built. However, they will settle for hard working, loyal and committed. Even the phrase, "Love at first sight," is skin deep, referring to the lovely face and sexy butt, not to the inner core.

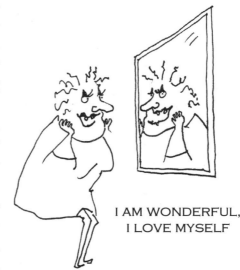

I AM WONDERFUL,
I LOVE MYSELF

Of course, someone who initially looks attractive can begin to lose that attractiveness as soon as he speaks. People who are not strikingly beautiful can grow more beautiful when one gets to know them because of the depth and range of their personality, or their loving kindness.

That is why it is important to strip away the superficialities, the shallowness of our existence, to truly see within the total context of both mind and body, not just body. While a part of us will always need to be reflected in the eyes of friends, family and lovers in order to have a reality base, we also need to cultivate self-reliance to select for ourselves the personal goals and personal path to self-completion. Too often we dress to please others, say what others want to hear, tell white lies to be polite. We become accommodating as we lose our self-confidence and our true identity.

When we look at the mirror on the wall, we have to see ourselves realistically and answer the identity question for ourselves. No supernatural voice will tell us the answer we want to hear. Hopefully, our question won't be, "Who is the fairest of them all?"

But what if we really don't like what we see on a realistic level? Perhaps we have put on too many pounds or become a bit flabby. We have the power to take action, changing our appearance to suit our self-image. When Michelangelo was sculpting the statue of David, he took away what David *was not*. We can exercise and weight-train our way to improve appearance as we create a positive and healthy self-acceptance, ultimately self-appreciation. However, beware of excess!

When I exercise in the gym and a woman passes by telling me I look good, I get nervous. I seek out my personal trainer and ask, "Am I getting too skinny?" I have observed that when women compliment one another in the gym it means, thinner is better. "You can't be too thin" is a popular comment. Anorexia, bulimia and over-exercising occur predominantly among women who measure well-being on a scale, rather than measure their energy level, happiness, or health. When women weight train, they tighten their bodies as they burn fat while increasing muscle mass. They go down at least one dress size, yet their weight might remain the same because muscle weighs more than fat! Even though they are thinner because of their firmer bodies, they evaluate their progress by the numbers on the scale and do not see the transformation. Instead, they sigh in disappointment that after all that hard work, nothing has changed because they haven't lost a pound!

And let us not forget men. While anorexia and bulimia are generally female disorders, men can also be anorexic. They are not immune to obsessing over their bodies. Men tend to obsess differently, though. They do strength training to build bigger muscles. For some men bigger is better and one can't be big enough. While women deprive themselves of food and do hours of aerobics to achieve a slim body, men lift heavy weights and ingest steroids to expand those muscles to the limit.

Both an anorexic woman and a "big" orexic man can be considered dysmorphic, meaning that they do not like their bodies. They have a distorted view of their bodies and abuse them until their appearance becomes horrifying. Female dysmorphics become skeletal while males become inflated. They have distorted what exercise is all about—good health, fitness and life quality.

Fitness magazines, trainers and physical therapists tend to label clients according to three basic body types: ectomorphic, mesomorphic, and endomorphic as well as overlapping combinations. Ectomorphic is the most lean. Mesomorphic is a fuller body with more fat deposits than an ectomorph. Endomorphic is what is usually referred to as full figured. Each body type can be fit and healthy in its own category with a workout and diet specifically geared to individual metabolism and genetic makeup. It is unrealistic to expect an endomorphic body to become an ectomorphic body and vice versa. Each is beautiful, healthy, fit and sexy in its own context. When you know and accept your body type, you are on the road to physical and spiritual well being. Exercise will sculpt and strengthen your body type to create balanced proportions between shoulders and hips making you naturally attractive.

However these labels always struck me as being far too stereotypical. The names alone make me feel like an alien from another planet—ectomorph, mesomorph, and endomorph. What each of us has to do regardless of body type is to combine an aerobic workout for the heart muscle along with weightlifting to burn fat and increase muscle mass and strength. The spiritual benefit is stress reduction, for stress etches unattractive lines on our souls and faces as in Oscar Wilde's *Dorian Gray*.

Regardless of your body type, you should eat what your body requires in order to fuel it with energy, bolster the immune system and keep you glowing. Deprivation does not work, for human beings are not creatures who tolerate asceticism well. Instead, we are creatures who seek comfort enjoying the warmth that comes from food. That is why those who starve themselves by strictly adhering to no carbohydrate diets, periodic fasting, or only one specific food a day diets, usually yo-yo in weight loss, ultimately putting on more weight than they lost! Not to mention the accompanying irritability! The basic formula still holds true: if calories *in* are greater than calories *out*, you will gain weight. Moreover, exercise can speed up the metabolism making it more efficient in calorie burning. Muscles burn more calories than fat, even at rest.

Train yourself to accept and embrace your body. If you want to improve, by all means work on it, but have realistic expectations. Eat healthy and follow an exercise program. If you love yourself, others will find you lovable. If you are content with your identity, you can then expand that self-love to include others, providing them with a passport to your inner world. If you feel attractive, you will be attractive to your significant other. Sensuality begins in the brain and is often transmitted by a look in the eye, a welcoming smile or a warm touch. You do not have to appear perfect according to an artificial ideal; rather you have to feel happy in your own skin and in your self-perception. While happily cultivating your inner beauty, you transmit an incredibly radiant and magnetic joy. Others are drawn to your happiness because they also wish to cultivate happiness. "Be the best that you can be!" Transform yourself throughout the decades to keep your body looking beautifully expressive as it ages.

All things should be kept in balance: eating, exercising, work and play. If you are full figured, then aerobic workouts are great for you and should be emphasized. Combine them with strength training two to three times per week to create more muscle mass to burn fat. If you are lean and angular, do fewer and shorter aerobic bursts, no longer than twenty minutes per day; instead emphasize strength training to build muscle mass, also two to three times per week. Remember not to over-train. A workout that lasts over ninety minutes is considered over-training. Next check your workout frequency. Make sure you rest at least one to two days a week, especially when weight training or participating in high impact aerobic classes. Muscles need to recover between workouts. If not, motivation declines, energy declines and protein synthesis decreases. Ironically, if you over-train your muscles, your strength decreases and you become irritable guaranteeing that people will steer far away from you. More becomes less. No matter how beautiful you look aesthetically, your glow, your aura, will pale; you will look depleted inside and out. Cosmetics and clothes cannot compensate for an unhealthy mindset and the face becomes its canvass.

An important mind/body principle to be implemented at least once a day: Do something nice for yourself that makes you feel beautiful and happy. Then do something nice for someone else. If you are not in a service-oriented profession, volunteer for community service. You will see yourself benevolently reflected in another person's eyes. And that is a much better mirror than the one on the wall.

Ultimately, how do you wish to be described: how thin you are or …?

MIND/BODY PRESCRIPTIONS:

- ◆ Do community service, any kind of volunteer work and commit a kind act to develop inner beauty by sending out positive vibrations to the world.
- ◆ Talk about body image with your children and listen to their distressing concerns.
- ◆ Don't compare your appearance with the most attractive person in the room.
- ◆ Reward your body with affirming and enhancing activities. Eat a balanced diet to feed your soul. When you eat well, you send a message to your mind that you are important and want to be nurtured.

MEDITATION:

Sit with your eyes closed. Begin your breathing practice with one hand on your heart and one hand on your belly. Visually tune into your body (with your eyes still closed). Really look at your body as though you were observing it for the first time. Notice what you like about it. Is there a body part that you are particularly drawn to? Maybe it is your soft curly hair, your deep brown eyes, your long tapered fingers, your big shoulders, or your glowing skin. How does that image make you feel? Take a moment to thank your body for this gift and for supporting you throughout the years, always being with you. Is there a special way to express your gratitude? Visualize what gift you might give your body in return like: a massage, an herbal wrap, or a warm bath with rose petals. Feel your body accept that gift and allow it to respond. Gradually return to your awareness. Sense your surroundings. Awaken to a contented heart.

In future meditations you will see more body parts that you like!

EXERCISES TO LOVE YOURSELF:

OBJECTIVE: BEAUTY MEANS BEING FIT, HEALTHY AND SPIRITUAL

EXERCISES FOR ALL BODY TYPES
COMBINING AEROBIC INTERVAL AND STRENGTH TRAINING

This workout is designed to be performed 2-3 times a week. Create time for yourself at home or in the gym. If you exercise at home, put on the answering machine. If you have a baby, exercise while the baby is napping. Often mothers decide to wash the laundry, or perform other household chores while the baby naps. Don't fall into that trap. While the baby is napping, recharging and growing, recharge the self with exercise. If you feel tired and don't feel like exercising, exercise anyway. As your heart rate increases, the endorphins will kick in and you'll feel much better. The same holds true for men. No matter how busy or how exhausted you are, set aside the time for a workout.

At first aim for a 30 minute workout. After 4-6 weeks proceed to 45 minutes and after another 6 weeks proceed to a full hour. When you are finished, give yourself a big hug. You will need a timer, dumbbells and/or bar for this program. Remember to maintain a rhythmic pattern of breathing. Exhale on the exertion phase of the exercise.

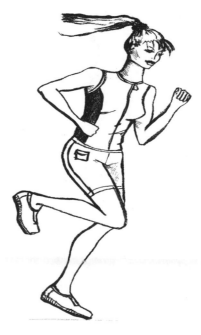

AEROBIC
Begin by exaggeratedly marching or jogging in place for 1 minute progressing to 2- 3 minutes.

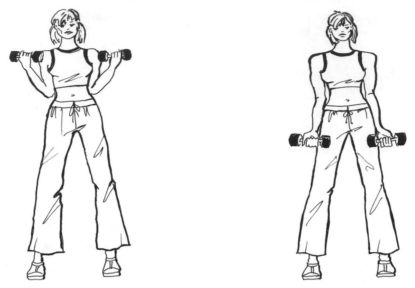

BICEPS CURL

Pick up a pair of 3-5 lb dumbbells. Do biceps curls 12-15 repetitions progressing in 12 weeks to 8-10 lb weights and 25 repetitions. **Remember:** *Do not use momentum; make each repetition count as though it is the only one you are doing. Do not incorporate the wrist, rather lift and lower from the biceps muscle. Always return to full extension and contract the biceps during flexion (on the way up).*

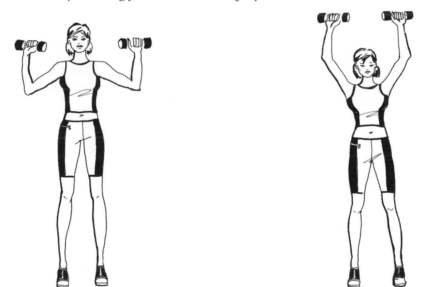

SHOULDER PRESS

Pick up a pair of 3-5 lb dumbbells. Do 10-12 shoulder presses building up to 20. As you advance in the next few months, gradually increase the weight up to 8-10 lbs. Hold in and maintain the abdominals tightly to support your back. Push straight up from the elbows. Don't touch the dumbbells together at the top. Don't rush (controlled movements).

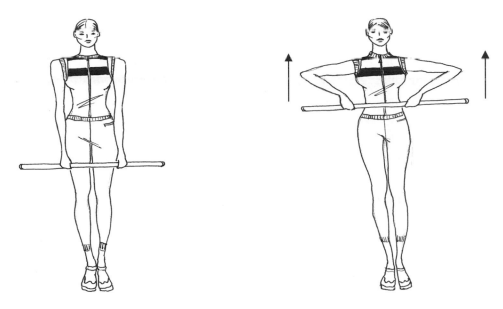

UPRIGHT ROW

Follow with a set of 12 upright rows holding the same weights or a 12 lb body bar using an overhand grip, lifting up towards the chin. When that feels easy, progress in 12 weeks to 20 repetitions as you gradually increase the weight.

TIME TO KICK IT UP

- ◆ *Do a set of jumping jacks for 1 minute.*
- ◆ *Then do a set of alternating (Radio City) kicks for 1 minute. Pretend you are one of the famous New York Rockettes.*

SQUATS

*Do 15-30 slow squats. When that becomes easier, add resistance and hold a pair of 5 lb weights vertically at your side. **Hint**: make sure your heels stay on the floor as you sit on an imaginary chair. The lower you squat, the more you recruit your glutes. Push off from your heels and hold your abdominals in tightly. Do 20 repetitions. In 12 weeks progress to 30-50 repetitions, or you can use heavier weights and stay in the 15-30 range.*

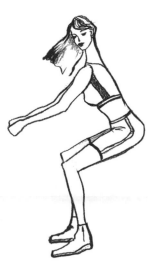

LUNGES *(Not Shown)*

Alternate lunges with arms reaching forward—right leg to left arm and then left leg to right arm. Stand with feet together, shoulders back and head up. Step forward with the right foot bending both knees. Force your body weight through the heel. The right knee is at a 90 degree angle making sure that the front knee does not extend over the toe. The left knee is bent to the floor almost touching and the left arm is extended in front. Keeping the front foot flat on the floor, step back with the right foot to the starting position; lower your arm to your side. Repeat with the left foot and the right arm. Do a set of 10 per leg. In 12 weeks progress to 15-20 per leg. For an illustration of a lunge please refer to Chapter 19 - **Training for Divorce.**

TIME TO KICK IT UP

 ◆ *Jog in place for one minute.*
 ◆ *Do one minute of jumping jacks.*

KNEE LIFTS *(Not Shown)*

Do 15 alternate knee lifts. Progress to 30 in 12 weeks and to 50 in 24 weeks. Remember to hold your abdominals in tightly.

MODIFIED PUSH-UPS

Do a set of 10 modified push-ups. Start by getting on all fours. Bring your body to your knees, dropping your hips while maintaining a flat back; abdominals are tight, legs crossed, heels lifted off the floor. Lower your chest to the floor by bending your elbows which point back as your hands rest alongside your chest, holding for a pulse count; then lift up again. After 12 weeks do 20 and after 24 weeks do 30.

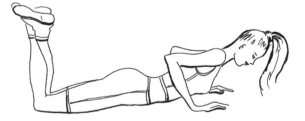

ABDOMINALS - BASIC CRUNCHES

Do a set of 25 crunches. Push your lower back into the floor with your knees bent and hold your abdominals in tightly. Support your neck with your hands and look up towards the ceiling. Contract your abdominals and exhale. Do each one carefully.

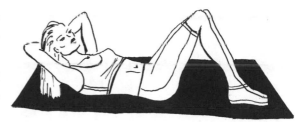

ABDOMINALS - OBLIQUES

For your next set of 25 abdominals, alternate right and left sides thinking about targeting your obliques (the muscles that give you a tapered waist); be sure to come up off your shoulder bringing it toward your opposite knee. Your elbow is your guide.
*Remember: do **not** lift and lower by using your neck. Do not rush.*

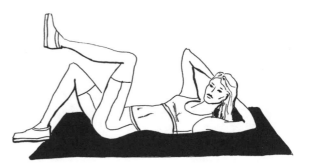

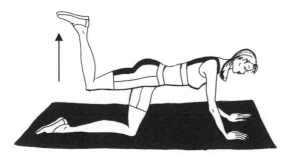

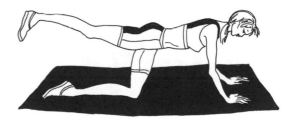

GLUTEAL LIFTS

Do 20 gluteal lifts for each side. Get on all fours and hold your abdominals in tightly to protect your back and maintain a table position supporting yourself on your hands. Then press your leg up slowly, knee bent, from the start position—a 90 degree angle in mid air, and press up. Note: this is a small move. Tighten your glutes and take the time to concentrate.

STRAIGHT LEG LIFTS

Do 20 straight leg lifts for each side. Get on all fours and hold your abdominals in tightly to protect your back and maintain a table position, supporting yourself on your hands. Lift your straight leg with a supple knee no higher than the hip and lower it almost to the floor, but don't touch. Keep those glutes tight. Don't use momentum. Think about each move.

REWARD YOURSELF WITH A GOOD STRETCH

For each of the following stretches, hold each position for 15-20 seconds and remember to maintain a natural breathing pattern.

TARGETS HAMSTRINGS

Grab a towel and while prone on your back gently guide your foot toward you remembering to breathe. Repeat on the other side.

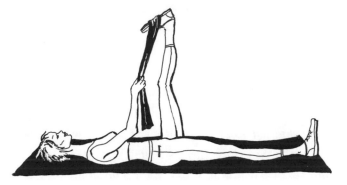

TARGETS QUADRICEPS

Turn over and grab your bent foot toward your back. Repeat on the other side.

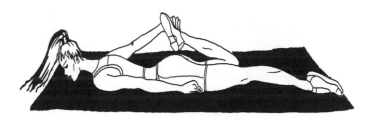

TARGETS QUADRICEPS

Balance on one leg or hold on to a banister or wall; grab your foot and bend your knee, gently tugging it behind you with your hand as you tilt your pelvis slightly forward. If you are able, lift your opposite arm in the air to help stretch your spine. Repeat on the other side.

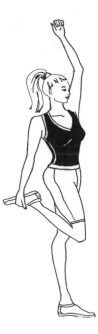

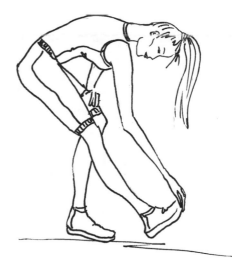

TARGETS HAMSTRINGS
Bend forward and grab your toe, keeping your leg straight, but knee supple; push your heel to the floor and sit back slightly. Repeat on the other side.

For more stretches for the upper body please refer to chapter 13, ***Training for Technology***.

Congratulations!
After an intense and balanced workout like this one, you are ready to appreciate your strength, commitment and vision for the self that you wish to be. No one can return to the past and make a brand new start. Anyone can start from now on and create a brand new ending.

CHAPTER 4

TRAINING TO DEAL WITH PEOPLE WHO PUSH YOUR BUTTON

No beast is more savage than man
when possessed with power answerable to his rage
Cicero, Plutarch's Lives

Anger and rage cause us to be at war with ourselves. We lose our veneer of self-control and then our sense of balance. The result is that anger dominates our thinking. Sometimes we do not release those feelings against the person or situation causing our frustration. Instead an angry internal fist punches against our abdomen, heart and temples. We damage our digestive system with heartburn and cramps and our cardiovascular well-being by raising our blood pressure. We create dramas, aggrandize unnecessary tensions because on some level we are self-indulgent, immersing ourselves in the stressful situation to play the lead actor. Then we replay these scenes reliving the original anger, keeping it alive.

When others push your button, what does this expression mean? Apparently each one of us has a special, personal button that triggers powerful emotions. As Ralph Waldo Emerson said, "we boil at different points." When someone, a boss, a lover, a friend, or a family member pushes our button, we are most angry with that person because he/she mirrors our own weakness. Even though the push of the button seems to come from an external source, in reality it emanates from within.

The question that needs to be asked: what about ourselves is making us this angry? What has disturbed the internal equilibrium? When we are enraged, we cannot think clearly. Our pulse becomes elevated as we grow breathless with a surge of powerful emotions. Depending on age and genetics, our rage could bring on a cardiac episode. Once we are caught in our personal tornado, it is too late. We do not know where the tornado will take us, where and on whom we will land, when the raging winds calm down.

Obviously, the best course of action is not to let our buttons be pushed: to stop anger in its course, and to move away from the unpredictable path of the tornado. However, because the tornado is unpredictable, we may be unprepared. We would have to know our weaknesses, the cracks in our spiritual walls, repair them to withstand invasion. That takes a lifetime. Also, new cracks in the wall are constantly forming just by living. It helps to realize that events do not upset us, but rather our judgment of those events. However, if we are unable to defuse the source of our rage, it would be better to channel it towards a positive goal. Instead of destroying, create.

Therefore we have to confront our anger and work it off. The mind has created the skirmish, while the body has to work it off for the mind to feel at ease. The excess energy, the adrenalin coursing throughout the body, needs to be spent in a positive way. Then the mind can be restored to its reasonable balance so that it can analyze why the battle was fought in the first place, strategizing how to avoid a war the next time, to win the next battle, or even to compromise.

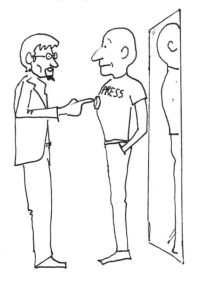

When we are furious, we need to imagine the self as a professional athlete who expends great physical energy as the mind evaluates the conflict. The athlete must function in a highly stressful situation, performing in front of spectators and facing the possibility of losing, which means not living up to the coach's or his own expectations. An athlete trains to evaluate the stressful situation not merely from a physical point, but a mental one as well. He centers himself through positive visualization and controlled deep breathing.

WHEN PEOPLE PUSH OUR BUTTON... WE ARE MOST ANGRY WITH OURSELVES

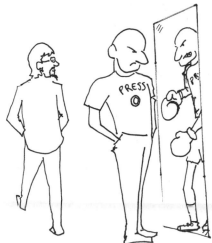

He chants a repeated affirmation that holds special meaning to restore balance and clarity.

For the non-athlete, as well as the athlete, walking provides a wonderful outlet for anger. Walking does not mean escaping, walking away from the conflict. Rather, walking allows one to walk off anger, gain control over it. As one walks, the pulse rate slows down; breathing grows calmer. The bio-rhythm resets itself and balance is restored in the body. One can think more clearly and analyze the conflict from a more objective perspective. It is important to differentiate walking from running. One might think that if walking is good, running must be even better, working faster to restore clarity. However, running is not recommended during a period of rage. Because the pulse is elevated, running will initially drive it higher even heralding a possible heart attack or stroke. If one is feeling enraged while running outdoors, the runner might be oblivious to traffic and obstacles in the road. Anger puts blinders on peripheral vision. Anger causes a person to lose communication with the other senses by dominating them. Therefore one is not alert enough to external danger when running in this condition.

After walking off anger, if one still has an unsettled heart, then boxing classes incorporating kick boxing and punching in a controlled environment will certainly help burn off the aggression. A good instructor will walk around the room checking proper form and precise movement. The participant must be conscious of each movement, in order to avoid injury caused by rapid successive movements using improper form. Also, because the participant is conscious of every punch and kick, he can direct and incorporate his anger more efficiently into each move, working it out mentally as he channels it physically. Eventually, he will realize at what or whom he is kicking and punching.

Weight training should be performed cautiously either with a personal trainer or a friend. Because when one is enraged, he is likely to lift too heavy a weight, or hyperextend the joints because of improper form and momentum. The excess energy needs to be burned off carefully in the weight room since concentration and third eye focus is disrupted by the emotional distraction. Ideally, one should walk off the anger before weight training. Then a controlled and focused strength training that would benefit the body, without inflicting damage on it subconsciously, could take place.

Ultimately, when the body is exhausted, spent from battle, a meditation would restore clarity and harmony between the mind and the body. While you are meditating, you could figure out what aroused your anger. Most likely, it was something about you, an insecurity, fear, or an unresolved childhood memory. Honestly acknowledging it would deactivate the wiring to your button. To *get even*: forgive the unforgivable and love the unlovable. This will restore your equanimity. Because forgiving the transgressor is one of the hardest things to do—in fact it is Divine; here is a suggestion: try to forego the incident or the words. Move it to the back of your consciousness. Each time you remember, you fuel the anger and keep it alive. Learn to forget.

MIND/BODY PRESCRIPTIONS:

- ◆ Close your eyes to focus on the internal self. Slow breathing slows your heartbeat. Breathe mindfully: inhale through your nose to the count of four; hold your breath for a count of two. Then exhale through your nose for a count of four, waiting for two more counts before beginning your next breath. Repeat ten times; notice how your anger has dissipated.
- ◆ Avoid overstimulation by reducing your intake of high sugar foods, caffeine, alcohol and nicotine.
- ◆ Bless the person who has angered you. Everyone makes mistakes.
- ◆ Chant a mantra: "I am restored to serenity." The mind will actualize the wish.
- ◆ Cultivate a sense of humor to reinterpret the hostile situation. Try not to take yourself so seriously.
- ◆ Be assertive, not aggressive.

MEDITATION:

Sit with your palms facing down. Begin your relaxed breathing practice, inhale and exhale. Close your eyes and take a moment to notice how your body is feeling. Acknowledge this emotion to yourself: "I am feeling anxious," or "I am feeling resentful." Then notice if this emotion evokes a physical response in your body; do you feel a tightening in your neck, or does your lower back hurt? Bring all your attention to the very spot that is tense or hurts. Breathe deeply and send oxygen to the body part that is in pain and allow the oxygen to relax and restore it. Now with your mind's eye visualize a turbulent sea. Go towards the edge of the pounding surf. Can you see your reflection in the stormy sea? Can you find yourself amidst the rage? Allow your rage to become the sea's rage. Notice how you cannot see your reflection; if only the waters were calm, if only your rage had dissipated. You cannot see yourself or your life clearly while the seas are turbulent. Now visualize a lake. Kneel down at the lake's edge and look at your reflection. The lake is calm. Your emotions have subsided. Notice that your reflection is crystal clear. Peer into the still water for a moment. Everything in your life is coming into focus. Return to the calm rhythm of your breath and your awareness. Your angry waters have subsided. You feel free to approach life with love in your heart because you see what is distinctly true. Open your eyes.

EXERCISES TO DEAL WITH ANGER: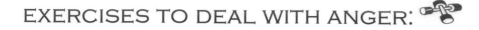

OBJECTIVE: GET IT OFF YOUR CHEST

CHEST PRESS

The chest press machine at the gym keeps you in proper form as you push away the anger in your heart. While you do this exercise, think or say, "I push away negative feelings of anger and resentment and open my heart to love and compassion." Keep your shoulders down and your back flat against the seat. Set the weight that is appropriate for you and push off 8-10 repetitions for 3 sets. Remember to keep the joints in your arms soft. Exhale on the effort. As you advance, increase the repetitions per set and gradually add more weight. Note: Never fully lock or stiffen the elbow joint.

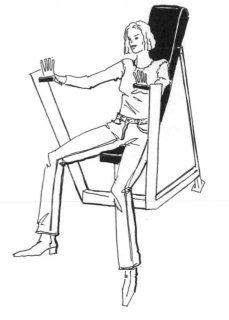

ASSUME A HORSE STANCE

Keep your *knees bent and abdominals tight - extend your arms out keeping your joints soft, let your palms hug a punching bag. Then squeeze your palms in hard as your arms extend straight, not bending the elbow for 3-5 seconds, working up to 10 seconds. Don't forget to breathe! Squeeze the anger right out of your body, so that it does not do physical damage by creating dis-ease. Try to do 3 sets with 5 repetitions per set, depending on how angry you are. For a more advanced move hold a squat position while squeezing the punching bag for 5-10 seconds.*

Remember: Punching is contraindicated! Remain non-violent.

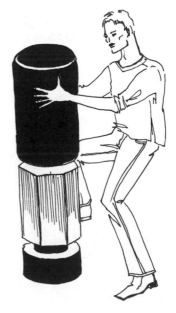

LOTUS POSITION

Instead of sitting on a hot bed of anger, try sitting on a cool flower. Assume a beginner's Lotus position. Keep the body erect with the head, neck and chest in a straight line. From an easy sitting posture cross your legs in a modified Lotus position. Touch your thumb to your forefinger to create a circle of good energy, allowing the negative energy to drain from your remaining three fingers, as you rest your hands on your legs. Now would be a good time to meditate on peace and serenity.

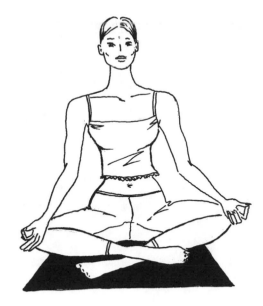

CHAPTER 5

TRAINING FOR WHEN YOU ARE AFRAID

So slippery that the fear's as bad as falling
Shakespeare, Cymbeline

Monsters, shadows, nightmares, phobias and death lurk in the recesses of our minds. We are exceptionally creative at conjuring up fears that intimidate and paralyze us from moving forward and flowing naturally. We are afraid to trust our intuition because we might be wrong. We are afraid to venture where our self-expression would lead us, for what if we are not any good, or what if we are too good. Instead, we barricade the "true" self with excuses such as, "I'm not ready yet." Our deepest fear paradoxically is not that we are not good enough, but that we are exceptionally powerful, so we shrink, or suppress our aura from other people who might feel insecure around us. In some cases we do not believe in our innate ability to heal the body when we get sick. We fear dying. However, what we really fear is not having lived our true life.

What are we scared of? Exposure frightens us, for it opens up the possibility of rejection or success. Therefore we feel that it is better to be contracted and safe than to emerge from the cocoon. We are also afraid to trust; we suspect others of ulterior motives. We are afraid to trust a significant other and reveal our feelings. Do we feel unworthy of love? We are even afraid to trust our own feelings, which would have led us to relationships that hold powerful attractions. We become frightened that we will be hurt, or that we will hurt someone else, not trusting that the universe has a training session in mind for each relationship. Usually, we are attracted to someone who will teach us what we need to learn.

What we fear in another person or in a goal, ironically, is what we need most to learn about ourselves. If we are acrophobic, afraid of heights, we are afraid of success, or at least feel pressured about remaining at the top. If we are agoraphobic, afraid of the marketplace, we fear sharing and exchanging ideas with others; maybe, we believe that we have nothing to contribute, or others won't like us. Some of us fear ice skating because we do not trust our ability to glide and find a point of balance in an unstable environment. Some of us are afraid to swim, to trust our self-expression in a different, more fluid medium. Afraid of the dark? We fear the unknown, the stage of transformation, known as the transition period. *We are even afraid to admit that we are afraid.*

All our fears point like arrows in one direction: the fear of living a true life, to be who we are. "What will people say?" Some of us tremble when committing to a significant other because we feel that person will have too much power over our heart and our identity. On the other hand, some of us fear living alone without a significant other and therefore rush into a relationship to avoid knowing and accepting the true self. People who are stuck in "terrible" jobs resist change because of performance anxiety to prove ability all over again to new authority figures: Too old to be given a "report card." However, the solution is intellectually simple, yet hard to accept emotionally: The person returning your gaze from the mirror is the one you have to answer to every day.

It all comes full circle to the Garden of Eden where God forbade Adam and Eve to eat from the Tree of Knowledge. And when they did eat, they left their innocent state to arrive at a new experienced state. They were punished for this first disobedience, releasing fear into the world. However, all that changed was their perception. It has become our spiritual legacy, this "crime" of seeking new knowledge along with fearing punishment. Perhaps, our eviction from paradise was a set-up, a necessary learning experience to help us find our own path. After all, in the beginning Eden was just handed to Adam and Eve. They didn't have to achieve it, or comprehend what they had. They just had to be. Each experience in life is absolutely necessary to move us to the next place until this moment.

Confronting our fears is the hardest achievement of all our goals. Our external fears are manifestations of the insecure inner self. For once we recognize, face and then embrace our inner selves, what remains to be feared? We become self-sufficient, fulfilling our own needs, leaving our insecurities by the wayside. For example, if a lover ends a relationship with you, it means your journey together is over. Your learning experience together is finished and it is time for someone new to enlighten you. When we face phobias, we face internal walls, which hinder us from living in greater knowledge and in joyful experience. As long as we were evicted from paradise, let's make the most of our experiences on earth.

Whenever we feel afraid, we could try to whistle or sing a happy tune as the old song suggests or recite the maxim, "The person who fears to do many things, does very little." These simple homespun persuaders are effective in alleviating basic fears, reminding us that happier times will soon follow. Any comforting repeated quote will work.

Fear pops up in the gym, too. Many of us are afraid to go to the gym, or take an exercise class. For example, an overweight person might feel that if he doesn't try, he can't fail. A woman might worry that everyone else will look better. Also, some women are scared of weight training because they believe that they will bulk up, looking like Hercules if they lift heavy weights. Another fear is being perceived as clumsy in aerobics class, unable to follow the steps. However, men fear the aerobics room even more than women. "I'll look silly." "I'll make a fool of myself." The best way to overcome these fears is to exercise with a friend.

Remember your very first day at school: how afraid you were of the teacher, the classroom, making friends, making a fool of yourself! Well, you didn't go by yourself. Someone took you by the hand, your mother, father, or older sibling. Similarly, a personal trainer can assist in an individualized program, gradually working through a client's fears of

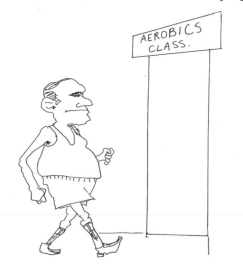

exercise. Working out with a buddy is motivating. If you go to the gym regularly, you will make "gym" friends who will take a class, or train with you. And if you choose to exercise at home, work with a personal trainer or invite a friend to your house to develop consistency and structure.

Similarly, when you are afraid of going alone to a doctor, a party, or a vacation, you invite a friend. Even in the midst of life's trials, when you feel like you have no friend to call and are frightened, there are guardian angels to take you by the hand and lead you to the Promised Land of self-realization and happiness. Hint: If you pray, or meditate, you facilitate their appearance. Also, do not expect the traditional wings and celestial halos. Angels may assume the form of a clerk, a hair dresser, or a child.

As for me, I would love to have an invisible angel help me lift weights, especially the last few repetitions. Lifting weights when we are afraid requires trust. We must trust our selves, the science, the equipment and the instructor. No one, from the beginner to the elite, is immune to this type of fear, especially someone who has been injured in a sport. We do not dive into the water before we learn how to swim. Yet we cannot learn how to swim outside of the water,

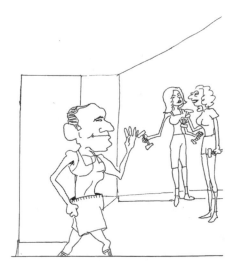

on land. We learn how to swim in the new medium, trusting the instructor, our bodies and minds that we will keep afloat. We take small steps when we learn. If we are phobic, we desensitize ourselves slowly, with aversion therapy. In other words, we confront the frightening situation, exposing ourselves to it little by little, loosening its grip on our spirits.

However, we do not want to deny our fears. We need to learn to handle fear by understanding that it is a normal response, a survival instinct, preparing a person for either fight or flight. When we deny the fear, which is often necessary to prepare us to assess a situation, we are unable to set up for stress. When we take a test or perform athletically, some degree of stress or nervousness actually triggers a successful performance. Visualization and breathing techniques, especially deep abdominal breathing carrying oxygen to the muscles, are helpful for taking the sting out of fear. Asking the self, "What is the worst that can happen?" Often minimizes the stress of the fearful outcome. We have to prepare mind and body to work through anxiety and channel the adrenalin surge to work for our benefit.

Worthwhile to remember is that with no effort in things, there can be no gains! At the gym, when participating in a team sport, or at a job presentation, review the basics to ensure mastery. Pump yourself up with positive talk; sing a tune that holds special meaning for you. Chant a mantra and positively visualize the outcome. Project yourself into the activity and picture your successful performance. This will help to develop your concentration to work alongside your fear, instead of fear distracting you from concentrating.

MIND/BODY PRESCRIPTIONS:

WORK THROUGH FEAR TO BECOME PRODUCTIVE

- Speak up and reveal your honest opinion
- Travel to a country where you do not speak the language and make yourself understood.
- Leave a party when you no longer want to be there.
- Quit your job if you hate it, even if you don't know what your next job will be and where your necessary income is going to come from.
- Ask someone who appears unattainable to go out on a date.

IN THE GYM:
- Take a totally new class with an instructor whose class is being videotaped.
- Run sprints after you have done many leg exercises using heavily weighted machines, like the leg press, hamstring curl and leg extension.
- Let yourself be thrown to the ground when learning a martial arts strategy.
- Fall back into your trainer's arms, trusting he will catch you, after you have given him a hard time during your training session.
- Jog: Run off your fear. As the endorphins are released and you feel excited, start to think or say aloud, "I can do it. I can do it."

MEDITATION:

Sit up with your eyes closed placing one hand on your abdomen and one hand on your heart. Begin your breathing practice. Inhale and exhale. With each breath, say to yourself that you are calming your heart. Imagine that you are walking barefoot on a foreign beach. The night is dark and all you can see is a bright moon reflected on a mysterious dark ocean. Look at the black waters. Can you picture yourself swimming in this dark sea? Are you afraid? Be alone with that fear for a moment. Connect with your emotion and feel where it resides in your body - in your heart, your head, your legs. Think about what aspects of your life you are afraid to jump into. Remember that fear itself is not an enemy. Detach yourself for a moment and take a close look at your fear. Do not judge it, but instead draw closer and try to befriend it. Smile deep inside. Perceive your surroundings as safe and secure. Imagine this sandy beach with familiar and comforting signposts, the kind of markings which would make you smile during the day. Use all your senses to see, hear, smell, taste and touch the landscape. Take a moment to really experience this place, to get to know it. Gaze up at the moon and see how it lights up the water. The light amidst the darkness inspires you with courage. Find the place of courage in your body. Continue to inhale and exhale rhythmically. Don't let fear hold you back. Approach the shore and dip your feet into the water. Allow the warm salt water to rush at your toes. As you begin to feel more at ease, gradually immerse yourself in the ocean to a level where you are more comfortable. If you wish, try to swim, or just wade. Feel the calm, gentle waves ebb and flow. The waves comfort you and relax your heart. When you are ready, return to shore and sand. Return to your body. Allow both fear and courage to accompany you on your next challenge. Slowly open your eyes. Realize that when your perception changes, everything changes. Don't be afraid to dip your feet in unknown waters. Let the light shine on a successful outcome. Repeat this meditation whenever you feel frightened.

EXERCISES FOR FEAR: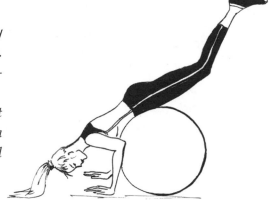

OBJECTIVE: TO FACE YOUR FEAR, VISUALIZE SUCCESS, AND DO IT

TARGETS CORE STABILITY

Balance your abdomen and chest on a stability ball. Gradually place your palms on the floor. When you feel centered, roll your head towards the floor and your legs up in the air.
Caution: *This is an advanced move. Try it on a carpet or rubber mat, preferably with a partner by your side, although you can't roll very far.*

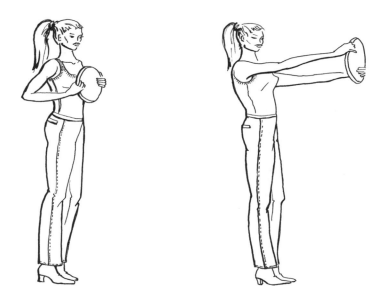

TARGETS SHOULDERS

Holding a plate (5, 10 lbs) press it to your chest with your elbows out to your sides and then push the disc out in front of you. Do a set of 8-10 repetitions. Aim for 3 sets. Next extend your arms, keeping your joints soft, rotate your hands to turn the disc a few inches to the right and then to the left as though you are driving. Do a set of 8-10 repetitions for each move. Advance to 3 sets of 12-15. This exercise can help prepare you mentally if you are stranded and need to change a tire by yourself—a frightening event for the first time. Your upper body will be prepared to use the tools in the trunk to jack up the car and twist the bolts off the tires. You will not feel afraid because the movement is familiar. You have used the plate to push out as well as twist and turn—a rehearsal for this emergency.

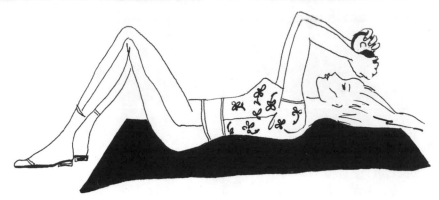

SKULL CRUSHERS TARGET TRICEPS

Lie on a mat with your knees bent. Hold a (3-5-8 or 10 lb weight) between the palms of both hands, shoulder width apart. Bend your elbows as you lower the dumbbell towards your forehead. Extend your elbows out as you lift the dumbbell. This triceps exercise is called a skull crusher and needs careful focus, so as not to touch the weight to your forehead. **Note**: *Don't let your elbows flare out; keep them in and pointed up. Do a set of 8 repetitions. Repeat for 3 sets. As you advance, increase the weight and do 12 repetitions per set.*

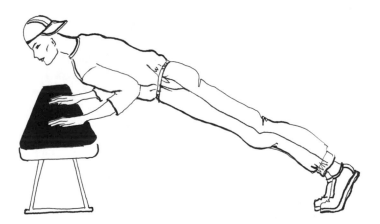

TARGETS UPPER BODY

Do a push-up off a table or bench instead of the stable medium of a floor. Hold your abdominals in tightly as you place your hands firmly on a bench while you extend your body full length with your body weight on your toes. Lift and lower bringing your chest to the bench; avoid bobbing your head up and down. As you keep doing this exercise, the fear becomes familiar to you and loses its sting.

CHAPTER 6

TRAINING FOR THE TIMES WHEN YOU LIVE A LIFE OF QUIET DESPERATION

Fallen flowers rise
Back to the branch—I watch:
Oh… butterflies!
Moritake

Even the sunniest dispositions can experience an eclipse. No one can live life untouched by anxiety, pain, suffering, or alienation, unless he is in a coma. Some of us visibly display our unhappiness. Others cry silent tears. Because we are all sentenced to die, some sooner, some later, we have to distract ourselves from the mortal sword that hangs over our heads, or the heads of our loved ones. We have the ability to transcend our fate, though. Some call it the soul's rising up to heaven. Some call it a noble mission on earth that sets the spirit free. Others who are more earth bound call it carpe diem or seize the day. Existentialists and students of Zen call it living in the moment and using the senses. Psychologists and artists call it perception and the angle of the light.

When a cloud descends and you can't see the way out of the fog, look for a source of illumination, a flash of light, the moon, or a lit match. However, the most enduring and powerful light is your inner light which never dims even amidst total darkness. Because we are used to being bombarded by many stimulating sensory perceptions, we find it difficult to see or distinguish our own true light from the extraneous fireworks.

When we retrieve our inner light, we feel immediate relief. A new perspective, a simpler, more basic direct outlook on life

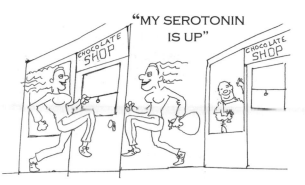
"MY SEROTONIN IS UP"

can take shape. We can't keep on changing our spouses, our jobs, our children and our homes, but we can change our own dynamics. Anyone who gets married and believes she can change a spouse, learns the futility of this plan. However, she can change herself and her response. Consequently, everything changes.

Imagine the wonder when my inner light greets your inner light. That's a veritable conflagration! We are social creatures linked by our mutual journey on this earth. We can learn from one another, share our stories, analyze them and transcend! We inspire one another to *conceive, believe and achieve*. When my inner light greets your inner light, we transform one another because we begin to see things in a different light. We grow from failure and from mistakes. From that dark point we realize small breakthroughs and develop compassion for others and ourselves.

How ironic, that without the darker moments, we would never appreciate the light because we do not fully understand or are unable to completely define an idea without its contrast. Would we really understand good without evil, or heaven without hell? The darkness makes our light shine more brightly. In fact, as the saying goes: all the darkness in the world cannot put out the light of one small candle. We become profound, more concentrated individuals who strip away superficialities to discover our inner core, at the same time recognizing it more readily in others. I would like to share a personal slice of life that demonstrates this duality.

During one of my workshops the program director formally introduced me, praising my various credentials and accomplishments. With a big smile I took the microphone and impulsively exclaimed, "Wow that sounds so impressive!" The audience stared at me as though I were the village idiot and wondered why they had come. Then I continued, "Anyway, these are not my real credentials." The audience grew hushed, eager to hear the sensational confession of an impostor. "I would like to tell you my real credentials. I am the daughter of two holocaust survivors. My father survived two years in Auschwitz and lost most of his family including his first wife and his three children. My mother slaved on a farm, hiding her sister and her true identity. My parents, refugees, met and married in Italy, eventually immigrating to the United States with me, their only child. Then in their later years both my parents contracted Alzheimer's." The audience now looks at me with pity and the sighs are audible. "Yet in spite of this dark backdrop of suffering, I see and appreciate the light. In fact, people are always asking me, 'What are you on? Why are you so happy? Are you for real?' Therefore if my father and my mother could create a house full of laughter and joy as they literally built a new life out of the ashes, then certainly can I who am far more fortunate. Everything else pales after Auschwitz, everything. However, I do not wish to be known as a survivor, or technically a child of survivors. I am here tonight to speak about living, really living." The audience and I bond. We trust one another.

Therefore do not be afraid to look directly into the soulful eyes of your sadness. Listen to its rain. Acknowledge it. Feel it. Dance with it. Confronting the shadow self is part of our spiritual journey. Everything that has a front has a back. The dark side is a spiritual companion to our whole being, and to our well being. Preferably, we might call it "the other side," instead of the dark side to avoid judgment. Anything about your other side that you wish to change, you can reform. For instance, if you are selfish, give to others in time or money. If you are alienated, join a community group, or do volunteer work. If you had an unhappy childhood because your parents did not love you, or abused you, then re-parent yourself, or better yet nurture someone else. Lose the hurt and the gnawing pain. Search for answers. Then when you have deconstructed yourself, lost yourself in tears and felt your pain, seek your purer, more creative, loving self. Let the raging waters of the past energize your present—positively. You have *to lose yourself to find yourself*. As Dr. Bernie Siegel says, "Lose the untrue life." When you find yourself, you will see everything more clearly, with greater illumination. Life will be more intense, more joyous. A brightly lit doorway leads to a happier existence to appreciate the good things with greater intensity. The cup will be half full, not half empty. You needed the contrast of sadness to appreciate the happiness. I have heard cancer patients say, "I'm lucky that I got sick with cancer. My disease helped me reevaluate the way I was living. I make time now for what is important. I appreciate the little things. I am delighted to wake up in the morning with all my parts working!"

In short, depression can make you more cheerful! No matter how long the hibernation, the cold contracting force of winter, spring and its vibrational energy, its lightness always follows. We spring into action. The winter has prepared us for the growing season.

Sometimes we need a helping hand to find our way through the "gateless gate" of life described in the ancient parables of Zen philosophy. It is hard to find the way, the solution, when doorways are not clearly marked and we feel as though we fumble in a maze. However, it has been said by artists and philosophers throughout the centuries that every exit is an entrance somewhere else. Go find a friend to help you see the way out. If you are a more private type, express thoughts and feelings in a personal journal. Notice what your body is feeling and where. Your body holds the symbolic clues and the key to the door. What has caused sadness to take hold of you? Why do you cling to it? What emotional rewards does it give you to have it drive your existence? If you have experienced a loss, accept and mourn it. Dying and losing are a part of living. It happens to everyone. Keep a diary and specify what you have lost as well as what you have retained. Just expressing your feelings in writing helps trigger change and points toward the door. Open it and move on. We are accountable for what we do *not* do, as well as for what we do.

Now strengthen your body to accommodate your new state of awareness. This is a perfect time to begin an exercise program if you have never exercised before. Raise your happiness index by running, taking aerobic classes and lifting weights. If you can control your muscles, feel each repetition, and image it properly in the brain, you can regain control of your ability to succeed in your relationships and your work. Let positive perception work for you. As John Milton said, "The mind can make a heaven out of hell, and a hell out of heaven."

When you have emerged from the chastening experience of quiet desperation, go out and help others find their way out of the darkness. Let your newly rediscovered inner light lead the way. When you teach others, your knowledge is reinforced. Become an emissary of sunshine; remember to smile. Just turning up the corners of your mouth releases serotonin. You feel better immediately and your smile will undoubtedly be returned.

MIND/BODY PRESCRIPTIONS:

- Draw the blinds to let sunshine into the room.
- Take a walk outdoors in natural light.
- Go to the park and push off a swing; be a child again.
- Go swimming; you'll be surprised at your ability to keep afloat.
- Play a sport or board game with a child to get in touch with your inner child.
- Do chin-ups.
- Look around the room you are now in and rearrange the furniture to help rearrange your perspective. In addition, you will release endorphins because moving furniture is quite a workout.
- Buy yourself flowers (particularly orange ones, for orange is the color of cheerfulness) and place them in a vase where you can see them. You will be surprised how flowers bring joy.
- Take as good care of yourself as you do your pets.
- Before you decide to do something, ask yourself, "How does it feel?"

MEDITATION:

Sit on a mat with your palms facing down on your thighs. Begin your breathing exercises. Inhale two counts and exhale four counts. Inspire life and expire the sadness in your heart. Continue to breathe and cleanse your heart. Close your eyes and see yourself go out into the night. The air is cold and the rain feels even colder. Imagine yourself wandering along cobbled streets with uneven dips and turns. Notice the chilling wind hit your face. What emotion does this environment invoke? Then you turn a corner where you see the sun shining on a green, lush countryside. The air is warm. Children play in a park as others picnic or stroll by a pond. Remove your damp coat and throw it away. Feel the warm glow of a radiant sun.

Your body feels much lighter and your feet barely touch the ground as you stroll. People greet you and smile. You pass by a balloon man who freely gives you all his balloons. What colors are they? As you grasp them, they pick you up lifting you off the earth to float in the air with them; your sadness has dissipated, no longer weighing you down. Look down below with a new broader perspective. Everyone and everything is smaller than you thought. You release the balloons one by one, feeling secure that you will not fall. After the last balloon flies away beyond the horizon, your feet touch earth again. A giant gold clock chimes: There is still time, there is still time…When you are ready, open your eyes to freedom as you transform into something great.

EXERCISES TO OVERCOME DESPERATION:

OBJECTIVE: TRANSFORM DEPRESSION INTO LIGHTNESS OF BEING

When you find yourself in a moment of despair, try viewing the world from a different perspective. Sometimes a physical act can symbolize or facilitate the transformation. The yoga Surrender posture will help you reverse your depression. Sometimes we have to be upside down to be right side up.

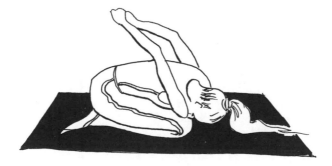

SURRENDER POSE
Sit on your heels. Clasp your arms behind you. Then gradually lower your head to the mat as you raise your arms up behind you. Do not force your arms to extend beyond a comfortable reach. Hold for a count of 5 as you inhale and exhale through your nose.

BENCH DIPS

For Your triceps; use your own body weight for resistance. Hold on to a bench, a chair, or any stable piece of furniture that you can sit on. Your hands are directly outside your hips and your palms face down, knuckles up. Keep your buttocks close to the bench and bend your knees as you slowly lower your body to the floor as you bend your elbows behind you. Let

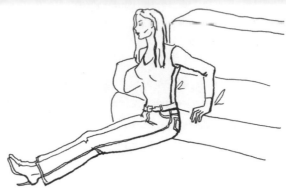

your upper arms and forearms form a right angle. Pause at the bottom; then slowly raise your body to where you began by straightening your arms. For the more advanced move (shown here) extend your legs out as you lift and lower. Begin with 8-10 repetitions per set; then progress to 15-25 per set for 3 sets; ultimately do as many as you can until fatigue to increase your endurance. Note that even when you lower yourself, you always rise up to where you began. You can always return to your self and your core.

CARDIO/TRAINING WORKOUT

A cardio workout is guaranteed to get your heart and endorphin levels up and lift you out of a rut. Jogging, stair climbing, bicycling, aerobics, dance classes, or any activity which causes an oxygen increase will help. The following is a suggested sequence that you can perform at home once or repeat 2 to 3 times in a row. There are no breaks between sets. Move from exercise to exercise smoothly and fluidly. Remember to hold in abdominals tightly, breathe on exertion and push off the heels.

SIMULATED JUMP ROPE *(Not Shown)*

Jump rope without a rope for 1 minute working up to 3 minutes. You can get fancy here: jump laterally, hop on each leg, or skip like a child.

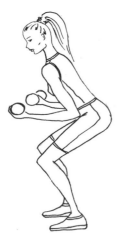

SQUATS, BICEPS CURLS AND SHOULDER PRESSES

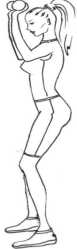

Holding (3, 5, or 8 lb) weights in each hand, squat doing a biceps curl from full hang to contraction and as you come up explode into a shoulder press. Remember to push off the heels when you rise and to rotate your wrists, so that your palms face out for the shoulder press. Begin with 8-10 repetitions. Increase weight or repetitions as this exercise gets easier. You push off and rise up in a victory posture.

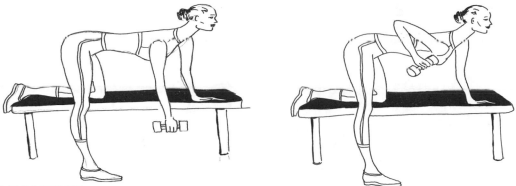

ONE-ARM ROWS

One-arm dumbbell rows engage the muscles of your upper and lower back. You can shoulder any responsibility. Begin with your right foot flat on the floor and your left knee resting on a flat bench or coffee table. Then lean forward so that you're supporting the weight of your upper body with your left arm on the bench. Keep your back flat and hold your abdominals in tightly. Reach down and pick up a dumbbell with your right hand. Look straight ahead to keep your back straight. Lift the dumbbell and pull your elbow back as far as it goes. The dumbbell is actually rowed until it is almost even with your rib cage on the side. Slowly lower to starting position. Do 3 sets of 8-10 repetitions on each side. As this gets easier, increase the weight or the number of repetitions.

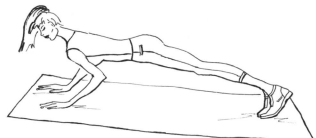

PUSH-UPS

Next do modified push-ups or full body push-ups (shown) depending on your capability: 8-10 repetitions per set initially. Aim for 3 sets. Support your weight on your hands and knees and cross your ankles. Space your hands shoulder distance apart, fingers facing forward. Hold in your abdominals as you maintain the natural arch in your back. Lift and lower your arms and your elbows bringing your chest towards the floor. If you can do 20 on your knees, then on your next set do a few full body push-ups where your legs are extended supporting your weight on your hands and toes, and then continue on your knees to fatigue. This exercise will help you keep your chest open as well as your heart.

ABDOMINALS *(Not Shown)*

*Conclude with basic crunches. Please see chapter 3, **Training to Love Yourself**. Lie face-up with your knees bent, feet flat on the floor and your hands loosely supporting your head as you look up. Curl to just a few inches, lifting your shoulders off the floor. Be sure to hold your abdominals tightly, pressing your back to the floor exhaling as you curl. Do a set of 25-50 repetitions. By strengthening your core, you can face any obstacle.*

CHAPTER 7

TRAINING FOR BURNOUT

Behold, the bush burned with fire, and the bush was not consumed
Exodus, II, 22.

We begin our careers with energetic optimism. We look up the ladder of success envisioning ourselves at the top. When the boss says jump, we ask, "How high?" Then our perception changes. The more rungs we climb, the ladder seems to get taller. The distance to the top becomes greater. Even the select few who reach the top, look around and say, "Is that all there is?" What do we look forward to on the job? Trudging to work everyday, we complain about the things we never complained about before. We feel unappreciated, overworked, underpaid and bored. We have a severe case of burnout. Therefore we need to rise from the ashes of our discontent to resurrect our initial enthusiasm.

One course of action is to temporarily leave the job and take some time off for a necessary respite. Some lucky people are able to take a long hiatus from work, a sabbatical of six months to a year; then return to their original job without suffering the consequences of absence. For example, every ten years teachers are encouraged to take a sabbatical from the classroom at half-pay. The result is an enthusiastic return with new ideas to stimulate student learning. After a year's absence the teacher has missed the classroom interaction, weary of having too much unstructured time; vacation gets boring if it lasts forever. Also, colleagues and students express how much they have missed the individual style and presence of a faculty member. Mutual respect is rekindled as individual talents and contributions are valued once again. The returning employee inhales this new, improved air of appreciation after having felt undervalued.

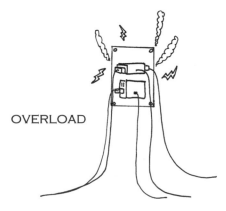

OVERLOAD

If you do not have the luxury of a hiatus with some sort of income, consider changing your career in mid-stream. Meditate daily to find guidance.

Creating the time to meditate daily will alleviate some of the stress and anxiety as well as enable you to feel as though you have been "away" on a brief sojourn for the spirit. Think about whether you have compromised your inner longings for the sake of monetary compensation and has this been at the expense of your personal fulfillment? Reinvent yourself. For instance, if you have been working on Wall Street, return to school and become a social worker. If you practiced law, become a landscape gardener and follow the laws of nature. If you worked as a plumber, study music and play in a band. Don't consider it a pipe dream. In short, start all over again; this time a little older, wiser and more experienced. Transfer your experience from one career to another. Work with a new set of colleagues or become self-employed to realize your untapped potential. Most importantly, do not become stale or bitter. Ignite yourself with new schemes and wild ideas. Don't limit yourself. If one scheme doesn't work, go on to the next. Don't give up. Redesign your ideas; connect with others to advise you or collaborate with you. There is strength in numbers.

If none of the aforementioned suggestions are viable, consider staying on the job, but refreshing your attitude. Continue your education. Visit other experts in the field and observe them. If you teach dance, take a few dance classes with someone else. Observe, study and learn. Then redefine yourself at the work place. Meet with your boss; communicate your ability to take on a leadership role. Do this by coming in prepared to initiate team projects. Have a plan for each new project you brainstormed and how you are prepared to lead it. Your boss will be receptive to your newly found vigor and probably allow you to implement your concept. As problems arise, tackle each one individually. Show leadership qualities by learning to compromise with the team. Appreciate individual contributions by nurturing personal skills. Stimulate the team, but don't annihilate those who disagree or differ. Instead, tap into the energy of contradiction and combine the different perceptions to create a whole that is greater than the some of its parts. Soon you will be heading up new projects, appreciated for successful contributions. You will have a new job without having relocated, making a drastic change in the work perception -- moving on without moving out.

If you experience burnout at the gym, because what happens in the real world manifests in the gym, then you have over-trained and over-exercised to the point of fatigue and depression. You need to pull back and relax. Take some time off. Rest your muscles allowing them to heal and grow stronger during this phase. When you return to the physical world again, change your workout program; cross train more often to avoid burnout. Sometimes it helps to choose a completely different activity or a new sport to create fun. Establish a balance between rest, diet and exercise to keep motivation high.

Use a variety of exercises to free your imprisoned imagination; begin by dusting off your high school yearbook and reading the caption under your picture. Note how young and innocent you looked. Note the lack of character and the smooth unlined forehead indicating there was very little thinking going on. Do you still have the same dreams and goals? I should hope not. Realize how far you have come and breathe a sigh of relief that you are no longer in high school with adolescent insecurities.

Next try to analyze what exactly you are dissatisfied with at the work place, at home, or at the gym, by making a list. Then write another list of what you wish you could do. Redefine your goals by writing them down. Once you concretely render a thought into words, it assumes a life of its own. It is your Godlike quality to make things happen. You create your reality.

Peer into the mirror. Do you look the part of the new role you are going to play? Get into shape through exercise and diet. Go shopping. Dress for success. When you put on the costume, you internalize the new role you will play.

Announce your plans to all your close friends who will help you accomplish your goals by reminding you of the song in your heart, not letting you back down. They will prod you, and at the same time hold your hand during the initial fearful stages of the unknown. However, once you have begun to activate your plan, you will become immersed in it and there will be no stopping you.

Become a child again in your enthusiasm, but with the wisdom of a schooled, profound adult. Now that's an unbeatable combination!

MIND/BODY PRESCRIPTIONS:

TRANSFORM BURNOUT INTO SPARKS

- Go wading or swimming in the ocean, the sea of life. This is a symbolic purification of your new self.
- Rest to establish an active phase of healing. Cut yourself some slack; everyone needs a break.
- If your motivation is low, check for seasonal triggers like the reduction of light in fall and winter and get into the light.
- Change your daily routine and break the pattern. Innovation stimulates and energizes both mind and body.
- Experience your environment with fresh sights, sounds, tastes, smells and textures. For example, see the various shades of green in nature.
- Learn something new every day.
- Change the message on your voice mail periodically.
- Change your interpretation of a situation or your opinion about a person.

MEDITATION:

Sit with palms facing up. Close your eyes and begin your breathing practice. Picture yourself wandering in a rain forest. Raindrops delicately cascade down dark green leaves. Stroll through a natural passageway that the lush foliage has created for you. How do you feel when the trees shake their wet leaves overhead? Continue to stroll slowly as though time is unlimited. Inhale the damp natural fragrances. Exhale your fiery breath. Repeat this breathing process three times. As you inhale, quietly say, " I am refreshed." And as you exhale say, " I release the staleness." You continue to explore your surroundings until you arrive at a pond, a quiet place. Sit and contemplate for a moment. Pick up a small smooth stone and throw it into the pond the way you did as a child. The sound the stone makes in the water is the only sound heard. See the ripples in the water. Notice how the ripples spread out gradually one at a time and then disappear into one larger body of water. Notice the effect you can have on your world when you make one small change. Take a moment to sit at the pond's edge and continue to peer into the water. See your cool reflection. When you are ready, remove your shoes and socks and dip your toes. You no longer feel burned out. Begin to return to your surroundings. Come back to your body and slowly open your eyes; you have a refreshed outlook on life.

EXERCISES FOR BURNOUT:

OBJECTIVE: HAVE A BALL AND CHANGE IT UP

- *Choose an activity that you enjoy. Go on a hike, play a sport in a league, or take lessons to learn a new sport.*
- *Take a spinning class in the gym. Although the bicycle is stationary, you perceive that you are on an adventure and your body's pulse and rhythm respond to your changing perceptions.*
- *Re-examine initial goals to see if they were too broad or unrealistic.*
- *Re-evaluate the motivating force of your work-out: Lean body? Endurance? Definition?*

MEDICINE BALL

Try playing catch with a friend using a medicine ball. Find a weight that is appropriate for you beginning with 3 lbs, progressing to 12. Push off the chest to work your pectorals and triceps. Throw quickly and catch quickly. Slightly vary your trajectory. This will force you to maintain focus. Begin with 12 repetitions for 3 sets, increasing to 25 for 3 sets.

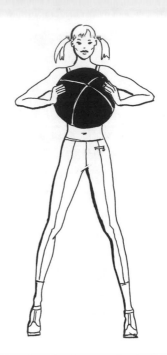

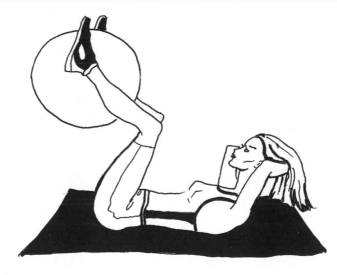

TARGETS ABDOMINALS

Lie on your back and place a stability ball between your ankles. First keep your upper body on the ground as you lift your legs with knees bent to a 90 degree angle and lower the ball without touching the floor. Be sure to keep your abdominals in tightly as your lower back is pressed into the floor. Do 3 sets of 8-12 repetitions. In a more advanced move, lightly support your head with your hands and lift off the shoulders. Crunch up as you lift the ball towards you. Then lower the ball towards the floor, as you maintain your upper body position. Repeat for 8-12 repetitions per set, increasing to 3 sets of 25.

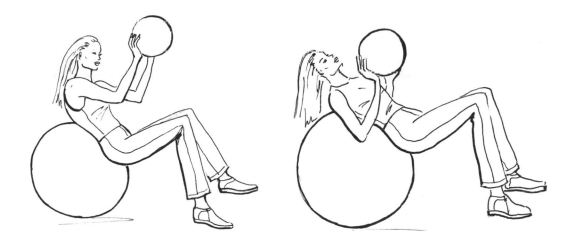

TARGETS ABDOMINALS, CHEST, TRICEPS AND BALANCE

Lie down on a stability ball to support your lower and middle back. Your legs are bent in front of you. Holding a medicine ball (begin with a lighter weight of 3 lbs working up to 9 lbs when the exercise gets easier) with shoulders raised off the stability ball, throw the ball to your partner and catch it. Then while holding the medicine ball, stretch back down on the stability ball to stretch out your abdominals and do a sit up off the stability ball. Keep your abdominals in tightly and maintain balance. Aim for 25 repetitions.

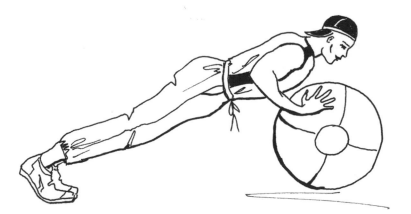

TARGETS CORE, BALANCE, CHEST AND TRICEPS

Maintain a push-up position off a stability ball for five to ten seconds. This is hard to do at first. You need to find your balance as you hold your abdominals in tightly and maintain total concentration. When you have progressed in due time, try to do as many push-ups or modified push-ups as possible.

STEP-UPS WITH A MEDICINE BALL

Step up and down a bench and catch a medicine ball thrown by a partner or trainer (weight of ball appropriate for your level) when standing at the top of the bench. Make sure to stand firmly with your whole foot on top of the bench. Push the ball off your chest as you throw the ball back to your partner. Do this for 8 repetitions for each leg. Then stand on the bench and lift the ball overhead and return to chest position for 8 repetitions. When you progress, combine the two moves: Walk up the bench. Catch the ball when at the top. Raise the ball directly overhead and then bring it down to your chest and throw it to your partner. Step down from the bench. Repeat for 3 sets of 8 repetitions per leg and increase the number of repetitions as you advance.

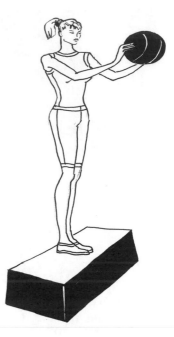

SIDE LATERALS ✝ SWAN POSITION

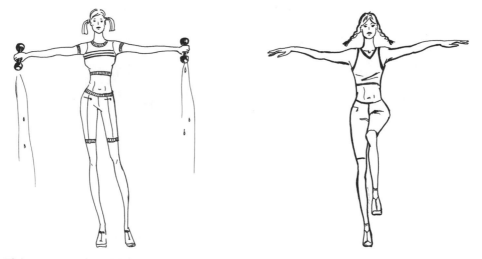

UPLIFTING SIDE LATERALS

*If you are bored doing side laterals, do this exercise while standing in the swan position with your knee up as you hold your abdominals in tightly. Always make sure that the head of the dumbbell points downward with your pinkie pointed up as though you were pouring water Do a set of 8-10 side laterals (3-5 lb weights) with the right knee up and then switch knees. Aim for 3 sets of 12. Please refer to chapter 1, **Training To Be Conscious** for additional details on side laterals and the swan position.*

CHAPTER 8

TRAINING FOR INSOMNIA

No small art is it to sleep; it is necessary for that purpose to keep awake all day
Friedrich Wilhelm Nietzsche

Since we are mortal, some of us wonder how we could possibly waste our time sleeping. As Americans, culturally, we pride ourselves on how little sleep we got last night because we were so busy! In fact, we compete about it, "Oh you think you didn't get much sleep, well I got even less sleep than you!" The boss is delighted to hear that we worked all night. No one ever brags, "Boy, did I get a lot of sleep last night." Moreover, we criticize overtly or subtly those who sleep more than we do. "Don't sleep your life away." However, anyone who has ever been sleep-deprived will attest to slower reflexes, fuzzy thinking, sad thoughts and overall physical weakness. Sleep rebuilds tissues and strengthens the nervous and immune systems. Sleep helps us sort out our daily ills to wake up feeling better about a new day.

When we close our eyes, perchance, we dream in symbols to get in touch with our subconscious thoughts. Often an emotional/spiritual healing takes place because our public, conscious defenses are relaxed as we sort things out unknowingly. While we may go to bed stressed, or depressed, we wake up with a better outlook and a new plan of action. Our muscles are refreshed; our internal rhythms have reset and our minds have sufficiently rested to integrate all systems. Sleep is nature's way of healing mind and body, even preventing disease by regenerating damaged cells while body processes slow down. Growth hormones for children are released only after a specific number of hours of sleep. That's why babies and teenagers sleep so much!

Unfortunately many daily obstacles disturb sleep. A poor diet is one of these invaders. Excessive caffeine intake is a stimulant, lasting for hours. Certain foods like bacon, ham, cheese, sugar, spinach, eggplant, tomatoes and chocolate contain tyramine, a brain stimulant. When these foods are eaten close to bedtime, we toss and turn and don't know why.

Ironically, daily upsets that we need to heal with a good night's sleep get in the way of falling asleep; we worry about them instead of surrendering, closing our eyes. And even when we make up our minds not to worry about them, we can't help but worry. Tell yourself not to think of a pink elephant and surely that is what you will think about! Paradoxically, we need to allocate worry time at bedtime to get it over and done with!

Sometimes a significant other snores loudly, keeping us awake. This causes us to consider murder with a plea of insanity due to sleep deprivation. And it doesn't make us feel any better knowing that the snorer's rest is being interrupted as well because his snoring is probably due to a cold, sleep apnea, or an early sign of heart disease.

Even thinking about falling asleep interferes with falling asleep. How many of us who get to bed late, or even get to bed early hear the clock ticking away saying, "Now I have only six hours left to sleep. Now I have only five hours, four hours, three hours... I have a big day tomorrow." The more conscious we are about losing sleep, the more frustrated we

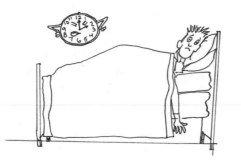

become and can't. Then the next night we worry about a reoccurrence and soon create an anxious pattern anticipating insomnia. The best advice: instead of focusing on falling asleep, focus on staying awake! Once again paradox works.

While there are sleeping pills, as well as herbs like Valerian and Kava Kava to help us get some shut eye, drugs and herbs can be habit forming and may cause us to wake up groggy and disoriented.

This sluggishness contradicts the purpose of sleep in the first place to enable us to wake up feeling alert and refreshed.

Some of us close our eyes easily enough, but awaken two or three hours later to linger in wakefulness. This interruption begins to occur with regularity as though we had an alarm clock in the brain to wake us. How quickly a sleep pattern changes! Sometimes our worries rouse us; sometimes our hormones are the cause. Many peri-menopausal and menopausal women experience this type of sleep interruption because of changing estrogen levels. When hormone levels are unbalanced, so are the mind and body. Doctors claim that even women who have regular menstrual cycles, experience sleep deprivation because of fluctuating hormonal levels. The more sharply and quickly hormone levels dip at the end of each cycle, the more sleep deprived women become at that time not getting the deep sleep necessary for well being.

When we are not sleeping or dreaming, most likely we will become depressed and lose our concentration. Every task becomes harder. We feel agitated about running errands, let alone tackling major decisions. Every glitch or problem becomes a nightmare. How do we restore our bio-rhythms along with our sense of humor?

First, stop obsessing about not sleeping. Figure out how many hours are normal for you. Normal has a broad range and is fluid. As we get older, we need less sleep. Utilize the extra time to work, read or create. How lucky to receive this gift of extra time! If you are functioning well in the daytime, you are probably getting quality sleep and are rested enough. However, what if you are not functioning well?

Studies have shown that writing down our worries, recording and expressing our problems in a daily journal reduces the anxiety associated with stressful events. Disturbing thoughts tend to play themselves over and over in our heads. When we put them down on paper, giving them an independent existence ready to be analyzed and solved, we close the book on those thoughts, feeling unburdened. I wouldn't recommend doing this activity close to bedtime, for emotions get stirred up during writing and might impede sleep. Having recorded these thoughts earlier in the day, we have the time to process them.

Next, we have to give up control, for sleep is all about surrendering and trusting. Our eyes are shut and our ears block out many sounds. We feel vulnerable to outside forces we cannot control, literally and figuratively in the dark, afraid we might not wake up. We say, "Look what happened to Samson while he was asleep; he got a pretty nasty haircut! And notice how long Sleeping Beauty and Rip Van Winkle were out of commission!" We need to tap into the universe and accept our mortality as part of the grand scheme of things. Once we permanently fall asleep in this life, we awaken in the next life. On the flip side some of us feel beleaguered by problems; therefore we do not want to wake up, wishing our earthly life was over, yet despite that wish, we wake up, unable to sleep.

Instead we might relax, ease up on our need to control, learning to yield and accept the natural rhythms of our bodies and life. Obviously, you can't order yourself to go to sleep, but you *can let go* in order to sleep. Forget about counting sheep. That's boring and usually doesn't work. Instead visualize in imaginative detail a place where you would like to be and where you feel safe. Go there every night and use your five senses to make it come alive. Fill your haven with images that incorporate sound, smell, taste and touch. For example, if you love the ocean, let your feet feel the warm waves while you taste the salt water spray. The sea gulls call to you from above and the purple sun sets in the horizon. Before you know it, you will be asleep. An added benefit: your imagination will soar.

Natural remedies can help us fall asleep. We need to change our diet, avoiding the tyramine rich foods mentioned earlier as well as reducing our caffeine intake. Absolutely, no caffeine in the afternoon or evening! Avoid alcohol in the evening as it causes some people to awaken in the middle of the night. Also, cut down on liquids at night to avoid that middle of the night trip to the bathroom. However, eating foods rich in tryptophan, close to bedtime like, yogurt, turkey, bananas, figs, dates, tuna, whole grain crackers and milk induces sleep. Sip some hot herbal tea like chamomile.

Another important sleep aid is exercise because it relieves stress, relaxes the body and heralds the need for rest. Exertion tires you out, especially when working the large muscle groups; for example, leg or chest muscles. However, don't exercise too close to bedtime, for the body becomes over-stimulated releasing endorphins and exercise raises your body temperature. Worthy to note: your body temperature needs to cool down before sleep. For most people three to four hours prior to bedtime is the cutoff point for exercise. Trial and error will help you find your optimum workout time, as many of us can only squeeze in exercise in the evening, after work and after the children have gone to bed.

Reading is a pleasurable activity that is sleep inducing, tiring out the eyes and the brain with imaginative participation in a literary work. The reader is transported to other conflicts and dramas, helping him to forget his own. *Note:* Sometimes the plot is too exciting, stimulating you to remain awake to read on. In this case boring is better. If you are reading nonfiction, or textual material, the added benefit of reading close to bedtime, is that you are more likely to remember it as sleep reinforces what you have just read in your memory bank. However, computer work has the opposite effect. People spend late night hours at the computer losing all track of time, passively stimulated.

But above all don't feel pressured to fall asleep. You cannot control it. If it happens, it happens. Don't go near your bedroom until it's time for you to go to sleep, according to your designated sleep schedule. Some studies suggest that the best sleep time begins at about 10:00 P.M. In other words, if you go to bed at midnight, you missed it! Try to adhere to that schedule as much as possible to achieve regularity—even during vacation. And if you can't sleep, get up and leave your bedroom. Go to another room and watch TV or read a book. Most likely you will fall asleep on the couch or in an easy chair.

Make the bedroom and bedtime a restful and soothing sanctuary. Remove any paper work, especially your work desk from the bedroom. Cool the room down as much as possible to help lower your body temperature. Establish bedtime rituals, for routine helps put you to sleep while innovation wakes you up. For example, try a hot relaxing bath about a half hour before bedtime. Have a snack of warm milk and whole wheat crackers. Lightly spray the room or your pillow with lavender or smooth a little lavender oil on your feet to relax. If you are a city dweller, get a "white noise" machine. Use sundown shades or drapes to block out early morning light that could awaken you prematurely.

And I saved the best for last: have sex or cuddle with a loved one. Falling asleep in the arms of a lover, or in a spoon position, will warm your heart and make you feel secure. Establish this sleep prescription with regularity. Your reality will be better than your dreams… You will wake up with renewed romantic enthusiasm, no matter how little or long you have been together.

MIND/BODY PRESCRIPTIONS:

- Drink a hot soothing cup of chamomile tea. Hot tea is difficult to gulp down forcing you to slow down, relax and savor the little things.
- Apply lavender scented oil between your eyebrows and right underneath your nose. The scent will send a signal to the mind to be calm.
- Establish a personal bedtime ritual that you religiously follow.
- Establish regularity in your bedtime, even on weekends and vacations.
- Get a massage.
- Give yourself a massage, especially your head and feet, with a little warm oil, using a gentle, circular motion.
- Chant a mantra: "I trust in the flow of life and I let go my fears and suspicions."

MEDITATION:

TO BE READ SOFTLY BY YOUR SIGNIFICANT OTHER, OR FRIEND

Get into bed under a cozy comforter. Begin your breathing practice. Close your eyes and allow your body to relax with each breath. In the twilight hours of autumn take a journey to a quiet countryside. Smell the crisp air. Barrels and barrels of apples... You have harvested and filled them all. In fact, the barrels are overflowing with red apples. You smile to see all that you have cultivated. Feel the happy tired ache in your body as you survey all that you have accomplished. As darkness begins to descend, your body begins to feel its weight. A pleasant heaviness blankets you. The skies are lit by a harvest moon and you are not afraid of the dark. Inside your house the embers of a cozy gathering still glow. There is a faint aroma of hot apple pie in the air. Succumb to the rhythm of the nightfall. Allow your body to sink deeper into that rhythm. Let go of the here and now. See yourself floating. Sleep is upon your heavy eyelids. You have taken care of each moment. You have taken care of all time. There is nothing to do because everything has been done. All is well...

EXERCISES TO INDUCE SLEEP: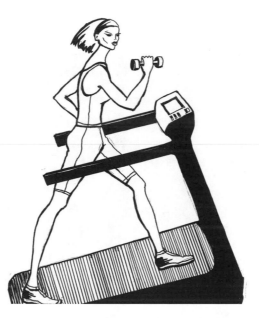

OBJECTIVE: TO WORK THE LARGE MUSCLE GROUP TO DE-STRESS AND PROMOTE FATIGUE

Warning: *Should not be performed within two to four hours of bedtime.*

GO ON A LONG BRISK WALK OR HIKE

*If this is impractical because of the elements, time, or personal safety, then walk on a treadmill. Walk uphill—this parallels your life. Begin with a 5 minute warm up on a zero incline. Then set the incline to level three. You may raise the level of the incline every 5 minutes until level eight. Walk for 30 to 45 minutes on incline. Keep abdominals tight to protect the back. Speed is determined by you. The objective is to keep walking uphill for at least half an hour, not how fast you can do it for a shorter period of time. You should not be out of breath while climbing; in fact, you should be able to talk. When this exercise becomes too easy, wear a wrist weight if it does not tax your joints, or hold a light weight in each hand. Cool down for 5 minutes on a zero incline and then be sure to stretch. **Note:** Keep in mind your maximum heart rate. Work in the 60-90% range of that heart rate. As you increase your fitness level, increase the work load. Train smart!*

CHAPTER 9

TRAINING TO RELIEVE PSYCHOSOMATIC PAIN

Canst thou minister to a mind diseased?
Therein the patient must minister to himself
Shakespeare, Macbeth

M any of us complain of back and neck pain, tennis elbow, chest pain, stomach-ache, or headache. Our pain can be intense, feel very real and debilitating. We start the day in pain and go to sleep in pain. We visit doctors, take CAT scans and MRIs; yet nothing specific is revealed. We take pain killers to alleviate the symptoms; then resistance is developed. The pain returns.

We need to believe and accept our physical pain as a concrete manifestation of emotional pain. Emotions provide the link between mind and body. When we deny or block our psychic pain, the body acts to remind us that we have not faced our problems. We might be repressing anger, sadness, or fear. If we are enraged and cannot express it, we might experience a stomach-ache, or a sinus headache. If we are sad and cannot cry, we might experience chest pain. Louise Hay cites in her books specific emotions that directly correspond to specific physical pains and ailments. In his books Dr. John Sarno discusses the role of repressed anger, fear and anxiety in back and joint pain. His thesis is that our physical pains distract us from

"MY LOWER BACK DOESN'T HURT ANYMORE"

confronting our psychic pains. In other words, unexpressed emotions rage in the unconscious. And what goes on in the unconscious mind affects the body. Dr. Sarno believes that there are three sources for rage in the unconscious mind: what has happened in childhood and never left us, self-imposed pressure to be the best, and the real pressures of daily life. All this anger secretly accumulates with the danger of a volcanic eruption. Therefore, the mind has the ability to shoot the pain to a specific body part that symbolically corresponds to the emotion to distract us from facing the spiritual problem, letting the true source remain hidden.

Many of us have a hard time accepting this theory. After all the pain feels real; it's palpable. It hurts! Some of us delight in an MRI that shows a herniated disc or a spinal stenosis. When a cyst is found or a calcification, we say triumphantly, "See I told you so!" However, none of us have baby smooth spines, or spotless MRIs. We all have internal changes taking place as we age. That does not mean, however, that our pain is caused by these changes.

Instead you need to face your rage, fears and anxieties. Begin by making a list of what bothers you. Next write a little story about what is going on in your life at this moment. After you have completed the story, put it away in a drawer for a few days and then reread it, noticing how your body feels when you read it, where the specific tensions lie. Even good things can create pressure and tension! Finally meditate daily to help dissipate the various pressures to feel centered and calmer. These mental interludes will gradually build up to have a cumulative de-stressing effect. By openly confronting unconscious anger its physical counterpart will eventually disappear.

Just as we try to create harmony in our relationships, we can create harmony between mind and body. Ironically, sometimes harmony is achieved through opposites. In this instance we can overcome physical pain by yielding to emotional, spiritual pain. Try the Zen way: become full of joy by pouring out anger and fear and accepting limitation without judgment. We can renew by airing out old internal pressures that rule us. Shout at your unconscious mind, "I know that you are driving this bus! I won't let you get away with it! I am taking back the steering wheel to get back on the right highway!"

Because rage and anxiety build up in the mind, the body becomes its canvas to express the damage. Upon speaking your mind to your mind, the body will naturally be better. Because there is no real rooted physical problem, perform the physical activities you have been afraid to do.

However, not all pain is psychic in origin. Certain physical pains must be addressed, particularly acute pain. For example, if you are hammering nails into a cement wall and afterwards are unable to hold a coffee cup, or turn a doorknob due to pain in your elbow, the vibrations to the wrist might have caused a *real* case of tennis elbow. If you are taking a step class, and make an awkward lateral move, which hurts your ankle, this is not an example of psychic pain. In these cases you must rest. *Active rest is movement toward good health.* Take care of the acute pain with R.I.C.E.—rest, ice, compression, and elevation. Straining beyond your endurance through exercise and normal physical activities will cause real problems later on.

If you confuse a real condition with mentally induced pain, you might create a chronic problem that causes the pain to last longer and inhibit your activities. *A doctor's evaluation is the first step in differentiating psychosomatic pain from injury, or disease.*

However, if you have checked out your pain with doctors and sophisticated scans cannot pinpoint any direct physical trigger, then go play a round of golf or take a yoga class. The worst thing to do with a psychosomatic backache is to lie in bed and stiffen. Loosen up by stretching and exercising. Stimulate blood flow into your muscles and joints through physical activity and deep breathing-- transmit positive energy. Feel the pleasure of exhaustion after a good workout. Pamper yourself with a massage, a hot bath and a nourishing meal. Release pent up rage and depression. Accept the positive impressions of your immediate world. If you become more flexible mentally, your body will adapt accordingly. Once the negative emotions have been banished, there will be more room for positive ones to be admitted.

And should your physical pain return, because problems and anxieties are part of living, you will have learned how to confront your pain and handle it; however, sometimes you will have to look to a new source of rage, or even an old rage with a new face. Bid that emotion to go. Assert your power and your self-love. Create your own personal affirmation to release past hurts. Here is a suggestion: *I create my own world. In it I embrace my body and my soul.*

MIND/BODY PRESCRIPTIONS:

- Have a daily dialogue, oral or written with your pain, ending with good bye.
- Get a weekly massage.
- Learn about crystal therapy. Try an amber stone to lessen your emotional load, or wear a ruby to open your heart.
- Use auto-hypnosis to imaginatively envision yourself floating, pain free in a safe, secure place of the past. Give yourself a loving, respectful suggestion. Practice this interlude every hour for two to three minutes–always imaginatively visiting the same place pain free until your pain begins to subside.

MEDITATION:

Find a comfortable position. Sit down or lie down. Close your eyes and relax your body. Breathe slowly with awareness. Inhale and exhale. Feel the oxygen infuse your body. Feel the toxins leave with each exhalation. Imagine a quiet, tranquil setting. Choose an environment where you feel nurtured and supported. Notice any resistance or discomfort in your body. Bring all your attention to that spot. Take a moment to reflect. Is there a symbolic message? For example, if your eyes hurt, is there something you don't want to see? If your back hurts, is there a load that overwhelms you? If your legs hurt, are you unable to move forward? If your chest hurts, what is making you sad? When an image comes to mind, it may contain your answer. The image may come in the form of a number, a person, a color, or a word. Don't judge your image. Observe it and let it pass by. Sense its ability to free you of pain. Believe that your body and mind are brilliantly engineered to heal. If you do not receive an answer, or have not been able to understand it as yet, be receptive, as it may come to you later in the form of a dream, or a word said by a friend or stranger. Feel at ease, as you let go and trust in your inner knowing. Allow yourself to float. Feel the ease and freedom of your movements. Tell your pain that you release the memory. Float over and past the pain. When you feel ready, return to your body. Speak to it lovingly: "I am here and now. I let go of the past. I can heal myself." Open your eyes and smile at the body part that no longer hurts.

EXERCISES FOR PSYCHOSOMATIC PAIN:

OBJECTIVE: TO RID THE BODY OF SELF-INDUCED PAIN

Whatever muscle group hurts you, make sure that you train the opposing muscle group in order to forget the original pain. Note that the new muscle soreness will be real and it will be good pain. For example, if you have lower back pain, work your abdominals. If your arms hurt, work your legs intensely. Balance your muscle attack equally.

If you cannot get to a gym, or cannot accept the fact that you are well enough to do the aforementioned exercises because the pain stems from stress or anger, then call a friend or your significant other who will smack you (not too hard) in the opposing muscle group. You will experience true pain and get your mind back on track.

For those of you who find the above farcical option a bit drastic or cruel, an alternative exercise involves stretching the afflicted body part with a significant other or alone by yourself if you are an independent or private person. However, if your significant other is the cause of your stress-induced pain, being stretched by him or her will help remedy the tense situation, providing an added benefit.

YOGA CORPSE POSITION *(Not Shown)*

Dead to the outside world, rebirthing your inner nature: Begin your stretches with a relaxation pose. Let go of the tensions of the outside world. Lie on your back with your legs shoulder width apart, and your arms in a comfortable position alongside your body with your palms facing up. Inhale and exhale through your nose. Feel totally supported. Send a fresh supply of energy to any body part that hurts, or is tense.

ROCK YOUR BODY

Press your back into the floor and bring your knees to your chest. Press your knees to your chest and using your arms to hold your legs in place below the knees, gently rock from side to side. You can rock yourself alone because you have the ability to nurture and heal yourself, or a friend can do it to you with gentle pressure, giving you the love and care you need. Remember to inhale and exhale through your nose. Do 5 repetitions.

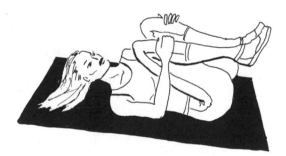

CHILD'S POSE

Do the yoga posture, Child's Pose. First sit on your knees. Then bend over to touch the floor with your head as your glutes rest on your heels. Your arms lie loosely by your side. Inhale and exhale through your nose for 5 counts. This posture helps you recall the comfort and safety of childhood.

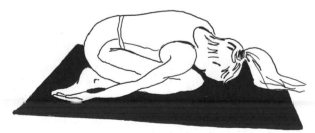

CHAPTER 10

TRAINING TO LET GO

He who binds to himself a joy
Does the winged life destroy;
But he who kisses the joy as it flies
Lives in eternity's sunrise
William Blake

One of our lingering childhood tendencies is to hold on tightly. When we were little, we gripped an adult hand holding on for dear life. What were we afraid of back then? The darkness, losing our way home, pain, abandonment? William Wordsworth wrote: "The child is father to the man," an apt saying as many people still retain basic childhood fears disguised and layered with adult verbiage. As adults we have difficulty letting go: loved ones who pass on to the next world, old relationships, ebbing careers, our grown-up children who fly the nest, and the earth when it is our own time to leave.

However, birds do it all the time. They leave and change locations. They push their fledglings out of the nest trusting that they will fly. Trust is the key word here. For we have to trust that when we let go, we still retain a part of what we let go. In a relationship there must be freedom of movement. A significant other needs to be allowed to fly freely, trusting in a safe return to the nest. When we try to hold on tightly to a commitment, to its original format, how we think "things should be," it can prevent the relationship from evolving to a greater depth. When we love someone, we do not possess; instead let him fly like a bird, who will return because he is free to choose—if the love is meant to be.

Sometimes marriages end in divorce and the two people involved consider it a failure. They cannot let go of the sting of failure as they become hesitant about future relationships. However, divorce is not a failure, just a learning experience. A specific journey has ended for two people who now need to continue their path separately in order to grow and develop. The original two people are not

YOU LET GO TO HOLD MORE

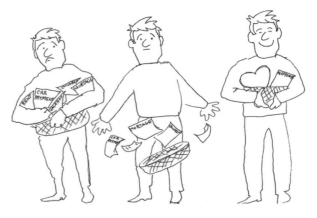

the same personalities they were when they spoke their vows. In any case no legal agreement can guard against change in a relationship. When we learn to let go, we can be true to who we are at different life stages. If one is always sacrificing and compromising his true inner feelings in order to dutifully honor and preserve the marriage vow, then it is only an external marriage anyway. That partner has already let go internally. One has to honor his truth and let go of guilt over what has been done as well as to let go of anticipatory trouble, what might happen. When we suppress, or condemn our feelings, we bring dis-ease to our bodies. My friends always tell me: "Stop over-analyzing! Stop saying, 'I think all the time.' Instead, try to say, 'I feel.' How does it feel to do this?"

Sometimes when we release the original relationship and the unhappy feelings associated with it, a divorce becomes unnecessary because a new relationship with the same person begins. We let go of resentment and anger making room for love. *Worthy to note-- an extra benefit*: *Disease cannot grow in a body filled with love and compassion. There is simply no room!*

However, we generally find it difficult to let go because we are fed a "restriction" diet of communal, religious and cultural values. If we always adhere to these constricting rules, especially when they negate our individual spirit, contradict our inner core, then we inhibit our life force. Like robots we obey restrictions because we fear shedding the rules that no longer apply, or never did. We are terrified about not doing our duty to others; we are terrified of communal reactions; but what about our duty to ourselves? Wouldn't it be better to let go of restrictions that contradict who we are? A Holocaust occurred in the twentieth century because of blind obedience.

Fear causes us to hold on tightly, specifically the fear of the unknown—"How do I know that it will be better elsewhere?" Often when we cannot release old patterns or partners, it is because we fear transformation, a solo spiritual growth. The love that we once shared does not die when we let go, for we can carry it with us in our hearts. We tend to look at the external shell instead of the inner core. Just because the physical presence is no longer palpable, does not mean that the spirit and the positive energy have disappeared as well. When our loved ones move away or pass on to another life, we may lose them physically, but not spiritually. Their loving energy and their teachings are still with us. When we let them move on to their next transformation, we fill their physical absence with loving memories. When my father died, I decided to dedicate a loving memory to him every day, remembering his words, his anecdotes or his jokes. I keep him alive that way.

Falling in love is one of the most beautiful and powerful passions. We try to cling to it, never releasing that fresh exhilarating feeling. However, that is impossible! Love is fluid, always changing, adjusting to a new circumstance like liquid in a new container. The intensity varies. Routine settles the romantic heart. Life's problems interfere; other responsibilities interrupt. Ironically, the more we try to hold on to that original feeling of being in love, the more we suffer its loss and keep searching to reclaim it for the rest of our lives, never to be satisfied because it cannot be recreated. We have changed. We are no longer who we once were. We have eaten of the apple and our eyes are wide open. However, we are still looking for the original Eden when it could never satisfy us the way it once did because our perceptions have changed; we are no longer innocent, but experienced. Therefore in an unhealthy way we become addicted to the original romance, the innocent idealization, the original Eden, the lover's initial physical presence. When we let that original intensity go, we empty ourselves of what is short-lived in order to fill ourselves with the next richer phase of the relationship. We make room for greater depth, for friendship and healing.

Actually our original passion thirsted for the primal energy of our lover's flowing spirit which cannot be held in true love like water flowing through our fingers. True love is an expression of Divine love. Our hunger for "true love" is our hunger for the Divine. We cannot physically hold in our hands, abstractions like love, energy and joy. They simply surround us and flow from one person to another. When we let go of our need for contracts, spoken vows and public demonstrations of love, we have attained the deepest love of all—the universal love that needs no testimony or pledge. That unconditional love is felt by a touch of the hand, reflected in the sparkle of an eye, or affirmed by a kind word. This is the truest love, the love that is tacitly understood, for when it is right, love gets easy access inside and out.

When we release our fears and our neediness, we make room for positive energy and Divinity to enter our lives. For example, my friend left his keys in the car with the engine running while he dashed across the street to make a quick phone call. As if trapped in a night-mare, he watched two teens hop in the car and drive off practically running him over when he rushed into the middle of the street to stop them. The police were immediately summoned, but they couldn't locate the car even though he gave them all the specific information; more-over, they had thirty days to search according to the insurance company during which time he couldn't even buy another car. My friend obsessed about the incident because he felt responsible and guilty; he condemned his careless actions. "That car is a piece of junk, but it's my piece of junk. I feel violated. It's all my fault for being so careless." He became sick with the flu; he had a relapse, and couldn't eat, sleep, or write music. Finally three weeks later he made up his mind to let the incident go. Realizing that unhappiness was driving him now, he gave up the idea of ever getting the car back and bringing the thugs to justice. The next day the police called, "we found your car and it's in tact." He was delighted, to say the least, and realized that the universe had taught him a lesson about releasing bad feelings of self-recrimination. He let go to retain.

Similarly, if we can let go of that old sad story of the past, as well as the disturbing percep-tions of the present, how much lighter our journey. Release the disturbing thoughts of the present simply because they are disturbing, cluttering the mind. "That person cut me off on the road to show me up!" How many car accidents have occurred because we needed to teach that "other" driver a lesson! How much easier, cheaper and safer to let go of the disturbing thought! Drive ahead in life. Stop teaching others a lesson to show them you are in control. Forget and forgive both imaginary and real indiscretions. We leave behind old disturbing baggage to be ready to catch life's abundance.

MIND/BODY PRESCRIPTIONS:

TO FREE OURSELVES OF INTERNAL CLUTTER

- Limit your suspicious "checking-up" phone calls.
- If you feel needy in a relationship, go on a nature retreat to spend time by yourself.
- If a loved one is suffering the throes of a terminal illness, whisper to him or her that it is all right for the soul to go. Reassure the dying family member that you will be fine.
- Release a balloon in the air. Watch it float away.
- Remove your wristwatch. Let time fly, so that you can function according to your internal rhythm.

MEDITATION:

Sit with dignity palms facing up. Close your eyes. Begin your breathing practice. Now imagine a long, long kiss—the kind that is composed of young love. Inhale the scent of your lover's breath. Let your lips gently touch. Feel the physical expression. Continue to breathe. Merge with its spiritual component as images, sounds, or words come to mind when you go beyond the physical. Inhale the spiritual essence of this kiss, allowing it to become a part of you. Be an observer for a moment, taking a mental photograph of your kiss. Now release yourself from the kiss. Exhale and let it go out into the universe trusting that you will never lose it. How do you feel when the kiss is over? What do you retain after you have let go? Hold the image of the kiss in your hand and study this mental picture. Smile as you perceive the love residing within you. File away the image of this kiss in your mind. Return to your surroundings and open your eyes to the love in your heart. Know that when you let go, you still retain.

EXERCISES TO LET GO:

OBJECTIVE: TO LET GO OF ILLUSIONS AND FIND BALANCE IN AN UNSTABLE MEDIUM

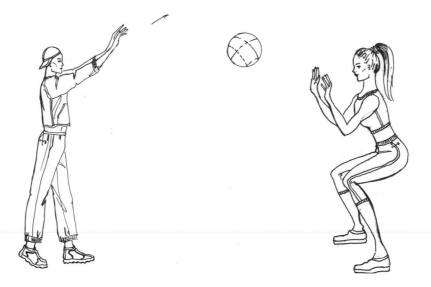

THROW A BALL

Find a partner and play a game of catch with a weighted medicine ball. As the game becomes easier, use a heavier ball. Remember to push off the chest. For a more advanced move catch the ball while in a squat position and throw the ball from that position. This will include the lower body and intensify the exercise. **Important:** *As you throw the ball, recite your personal affirmation about what you wish to let go.*

CORE BALANCE

Sit on a stability ball and hold your abdominals in tightly. Find your balance and lift one knee up and extend your arms out. Hold this position for 10 seconds. Then switch legs. Do 3 sets of 8 repetitions. For a more advanced move: extend the leg fully (not shown) and maintain stability. This core training move will help stabilize your body as you gradually begin to lift off the ground.

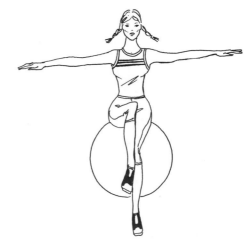

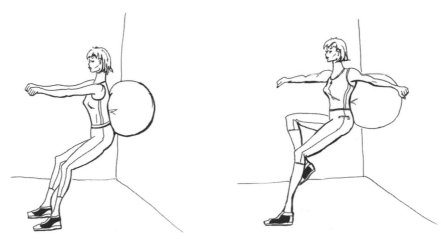

ONE-LEGGED SQUATS

Position yourself against the wall with a stability ball to support your back. Your arms are extended out and your knees are bent in a squat. Take it down as though you were sitting on an imaginary chair. Do 3 sets of 10 squats. Remember to push off your heels as you rise to start position. When this becomes easy, try to let go by doing one-legged squats. Do as many as you can, first on one side and then on the other. When you adapt to the exercise, aim for 3 sets of 8 repetitions.

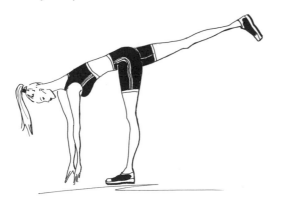

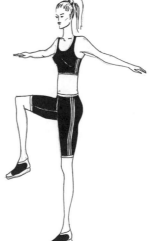

FLOWING STABILIZATION

From a standing position lower your head and chest towards the floor as your hands gently touch it while simultaneously your right leg extends up behind you. Do this part slowly and with great concentration to maintain balance. Let your right leg and arms flow while your left leg firmly stabilizes and supports your body. Tighten your glutes. Then slowly returning toward the start position, but not completing it, let your right leg come up in a knee lift forward as your arms gracefully extend out shoulder height. Hold for 5 seconds. Slowly put your arms down at your side and your right knee down next to the left. Repeat on the other side. Try to do as many as you can. Aim for 5-8 on each side. Hint: Don't do this after an intense leg workout. Your legs will be too fatigued to flow through the movement and maintain balance. Remember to breathe. This exercise helps to train you to let go deep within.

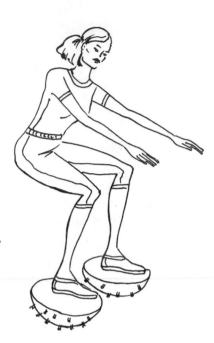

STABILITY DISCS

Find your balance in an unstable medium on two air blown stability discs. Hold in abdominals tightly, find a focal point and recruit your core to maintain control. Don't forget to breathe. Then when you feel ready, squat as though you were sitting on an imaginary chair. Lift and lower doing as many squats as you can without toppling. Gradually increase to 3 sets of 10. For a more advanced move, do squats on one disc. When that becomes easy, for the ultimate letting go experience, maintain your balance by lifting one leg in a knee bend as arms extend out.

Remember to keep those abdominals tight.

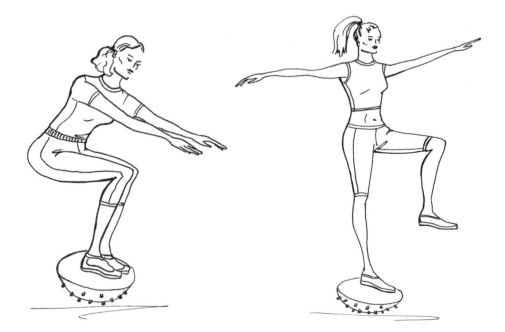

CHAPTER 11

TRAINING TO HAVE FUN

A little fun, to match the sorrow
Of each day's growing — and so, good-morrow!
George Louis Palmella

Fun conjures up memories of childlike delight: merry go rounds, playgrounds, ice-cream sundaes, pretending and the circus. Then we are forced to go to school, go to work and live with significant others. The fun seems to be sucked right out of our souls by daily problems and drudgeries. The process begins in elementary school where every child sits with eyes facing the authoritarian teacher at the front of the room. The child conforms to the rules and assignments as comments and grades erode self-confidence. School becomes a gated prison, a place of judgment where mediocrity often rules. Many children internalize a teacher's label, "I can't write," or "I have no head for math." Performance anxiety causes some children to develop nervous stomachs, asthmatic attacks and headaches. Nevertheless rushing to the rescue is always a child's favorite subject, recess, along with a child's innate, endless capacity for fun… drawing cartoons in class and daydreaming. Fun is recognized by a smile and a giggle, which physicians claim is the best medicine for reducing pain, stress and blood pressure as well as curing disease. Fun boosts the immune system to prevent illness.

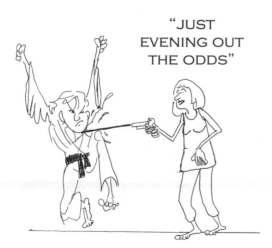

"JUST EVENING OUT THE ODDS"

Adults are emotional by-products of the school system and high parental expectation with the added stress of the workplace. Sometimes we perceive that supervisors make demands on us for their personal gain instead of guiding our careers and giving us the deserved credit for a job well done. We feel used, unappreciated and stuck. Even the best jobs, the most autonomous jobs, the most creative jobs eventually become routine, losing their original luster. Yet there are always "those people" who manage to have fun no matter what they are doing. They bring "recess" into their lives. Those people range from factory workers on assembly lines to pediatricians during strep and flu season. How do they preserve their original childlike delight?

One quality that enables fun lovers to persevere amidst the mundane or while under pressure is a sense of humor. Wit also goes a long way to defuse volatile situations. Laughter reduces stress by releasing serotonin. My children's pediatrician often alleviated the tension of a screaming, flailing baby who was getting a shot with an impromptu remark like, "Some days I feel like I practice veterinary medicine." We both laughed, but not the baby.

At the work place it takes two to argue or be bitter. If one of us is witty, or visualizes a nasty supervisor stripped to his underwear, a sunny smile inevitably breaks out in the storm, stopping the tirade. At the work place you can always re-tell jokes you have heard, or make up spontaneous ones to amuse yourself and others. Typically, men like to re-tell jokes, while women tend to be spontaneous. Begin to cultivate a humorous "eye." Notice the funny things happening around you like those recorded in the Metropolitan Diary in the New York Times. Personal entertainment is self-perpetuated and can alleviate boredom or hostility. The more you try to be funny, the funnier you will become. Your surroundings will strike you as amusing. Before you know it, you will be having fun and others will find you entertaining and cheerful. Laughter is contagious.

Another suggestion for having fun at the work place, especially if your job is robot-like, is to amuse yourself mentally while you perform the physical or the routine. For example, an older friend of mine worked for Tasty Bread many years ago. He used to stuff bread into plastic bags. I asked him how he did not go insane from the routine. "Quite simply," he explained, "by creating poetry in my head as I did it. At night I would come home and write down what I had composed during work. Any other job would have used up my mind, tired me out, blocking my creativity." Since his job was so-called mindless, he used it as an opportunity to create what he really loved doing. In fact he published his poetry.

So much for the workplace, but what about family life that can become routine and dull? After being together for years, couples who are able to finish each other's sentences and need a few drinks to go to bed with each other have lost their sense of fun. Once again a sense of humor is helpful in creating a playful atmosphere. Practical jokes, riddles and costumes create elements of childlike surprise. One could take a few lessons from British farce! Don't be afraid to be silly! Use any tools available, toys like a water gun, or a hat. Be unpredictable!

If your significant other is tuned into a sport event and you feel ignored, don't ruin his fun by demanding attention. Instead, bet which team will win and the winner gets his or her sexual fantasy fulfilled. The outcome will become just as exciting to you as it will to him! In fact, he will be eager for the game to be over to let the bedroom games begin, especially if he wins the bet!

Don't be afraid to fantasize with your significant other; view him or her as your playmate. The idea is *to want what you have!* For example, go to a restaurant and pretend to meet for the first time. Really look at your "date" from a new angle and recreate the reason you were first attracted to each other. Have fun! Hunt him or her like rare quarry. Use creative dialogue. Go dancing and let the music transport you imaginatively as music is a great persuader. Since a drumbeat corresponds to a heartbeat, ask your lover if his or her heart beats for you. Then when you leave together, arrive to an already decorated bedroom with candles and love notes. Tease out the lover in your sweetie. Tickling is particularly effective, as is a pillow fight.

Play sports together. Contact sports are even better! Go to the gym and train together to get your endorphins up, as well as your libido. Training together is fun, healthy and sensual. Also, most people feel better about themselves and their bodies after a workout. This translates to a better experience between the sheets. Exercise increases blood flow to the sexual organs; how convenient to have your significant other with you when that happens…

Go hiking in the woods or take a walk together on the beach. Natural fun is spontaneous and relaxing. Carry a picnic lunch or dinner with foods that are fun for the two of you. Some foods may be associated with good memories, or be symbolic of your relationship. For example, perhaps, your honey squirted ketchup on your shirt the first time you had dinner together. While she felt embarrassed and anxious that you would never call her again, ironically, you laughed and fell in love with her. Or perhaps, you met for the first time when you both simultaneously ordered the last soft pretzel from the outdoor vendor and ended up sharing more than just a snack. After your picnic, inhale the fresh air and look into each other's eyes. Then at the very moment when you hold each other in a penetrating gaze, burst into a run. Dare your significant other to catch you as you sprint. However, remember this is not a competitive run; it is important to get caught!

Sexual fun and games are all very good. However, if you lack a partner, or your partner is working all the time, or you cannot establish a regular workout schedule of at least three to four times a week for the two of you, then return to the regimen of the gym and make your own fun.

However, in the gym many people do not exercise regularly because they complain, "It's just not fun, anymore." After awhile a treadmill goes nowhere; an elliptical machine has lost its individuality, and you know all the choreography in your aerobics classes, for you can do the steps with your eyes closed while you compose a shopping list in your head. A fun alternative is joining a sports league or a team. Playing in a league or as part of a team requires you to be quick, competitive, and skillful. Typically, you exercise more intensely and for a longer period of time than in a gym workout, but you don't sense it because you are having fun.

Also, playing a sport uses more muscle groups simultaneously. That causes you to build endurance, coordination, balance and realize muscle function. Muscles assume another meaning, other than appearance. They can help you win. Also, sports such as tennis, basketball or volleyball incorporate abrupt stopping and starting, which stimulate both the mind and the body. Sports movements tend to be explosive, shocking the body into physical changes that promote a leaner, more muscular appearance. Physical fitness professionals recommend cross training or changing up a weight lifting routine to increase strength and reshape the body. In a team sport one never knows what comes his way. Change is guaranteed.

Most importantly, team sports allow the participants *to play*. You make friends, run around, get your endorphins up and stimulate your mind with new skills and challenges.

MIND/BODY PRESCRIPTIONS:

TO FEEL HAPPY

- Whatever exercise you choose to do whether it's running, stair climbing, participating in an aerobics class, or lifting weights, perceive the workout as fun. Don't worry about your appearance. Enjoy it! Listen to music!
- Skip and run to your next destination in childlike abandon.
- Dress up in a costume to try on a new identity.
- Buy a wig in a different hair color and length from your own hair.
- Everyday do something impulsive that makes you feel happy.
- Read a joke book.
- Watch more comedies.
- Bake a cake or cookies.
- At the gym give your personal trainer a workout! Reverse the roles!
- When you are in the midst of using your third eye focus during a training session, in a serious voice ask your trainer if he is "certifiable."
- Do a martial arts workout, but bring a water gun to even the odds.
- When your instructor starts speaking in technical terms using Latin phrases, or lengthy anatomical descriptions of muscles, demonstrate your own knowledge. For example when he explains that the workout will target abductors, insert your own in-depth knowledge of conductors.
- When your trainer does a workout for back muscles, request specific exercises for your dorsal fin.

MEDITATION:

Lie down with palms facing up. Take in a deep cleansing breath. Allow your body to sink into the floor. Close your eyes and breathe deeply until your body feels relaxed. Look up towards your eyebrows with your eyes closed. In your mind's eye, the space between your eyebrows, envision a joyous moment. Are you singing in a famous concert hall? Are you receiving the Nobel Prize for your discovery? Are you getting married in a beautiful cathedral? Let all the specific details take shape. Use your five senses and be there for the full experience. Hear the music and smell the fragrance. Come back to your breath. Inhale the fun; exhale the mundane. Fully participate in your fantasy. Experience the emotions that come up for you and locate them in your body. Do not resist. Allow yourself to be present in your joyous moment. Believe that you have the power to shape your destiny. Slowly, return to your original surroundings. Open your eyes and smile. When you return to your reality, recreate the fun by playing it out first in your mind. Then bring it out in the physical world. You will intuitively know how.

EXERCISES TO HAVE FUN:

OBJECTIVE: TO FEEL FREE TO HAVE FUN

If you feel like your workouts have fallen into a rut, try changing up the basics. Change frequently to prevent boredom and to shock your body into new growth. Consider sprinting in relay races and free style dancing to music.

1. GET INTO A GENIE POSITION
2. MAKE A WISH
3. IT WILL COME TRUE

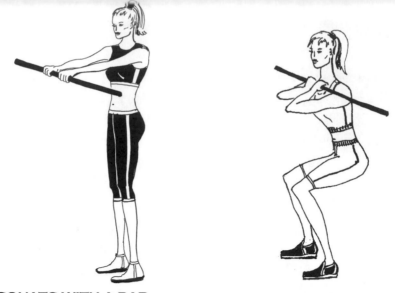

GENIE SQUATS WITH A BAR

Grasp a broom or a weighted body bar (if you are more advanced) with an overhand grip. Stand up straight feet shoulder width apart and squat pushing your glutes back as though you are sitting in an imaginary chair. Next, position the bar to rest on your front deltoid, supporting it with your fists and do 8 low squats without rising. Remember to push off your heels as you rise to the start position. Do 3 sets. As this gets easier, increase the number of repetitions per set. Squatting low provides an extra burn for the glutes while the bar provides extra weight to add cardiac intensity.

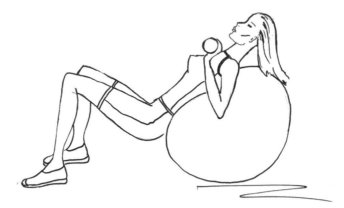

CHEST PRESS

Have fun with a chest press while you recruit core balance. Position yourself on a colorful stability ball to support your back and shoulders while you hold 2 dumbbells in hand (3,5,8,10, or 12 lb weights according to your ability). Joyously press the weights up to a point over your upper chest, palms facing forward. Lower the weights slowly, pausing briefly at the bottom position, then drive the weights back up. Inhale as you lower the weights and exhale as you lift. Do 3 sets of 10-12. As this becomes easy, use heavier dumbbells and execute 8-10 repetitions per set. Pushing off your chest and feeling supported helps liberate the heavy heart within.

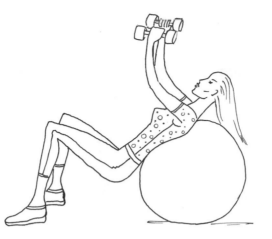

FLYES

*Ordinary flyes can be tedious, but if you want your pectorals to look full and round this exercise is for you. To create some fun, lie back with shoulders positioned on a colorful stability ball and imagine that you are ready for take off. Holding 2 dumbbells (weight according to ability), begin with your arms up in front of you and note that elbows are bent throughout this exercise. Visualize that you are hugging a giant tree. Then let your elbows come down guiding the dumbbells in an arc out to the sides. Slowly bring the weights up in an arc over your chest. Do 3 sets of 8. As you progress, increase the weight and perform your repetitions. Be careful not to hyperextend the elbows and stress the shoulders. **Visualize:** Flyes open your arms wide to reveal your heart, creating receptiveness for joy, goodness and love.*

SQUAT, CATCH AND BEYOND

From squatting to playing catch, you have done it all. Why not for the sake of change combine the two moves and add a squad thrust (not shown)! Squat while catching a weighted medicine ball, weight to be determined by you. As you rise, push the ball off your chest and throw it back. Then get down in a low squat position, kick it out on all fours into a push-up position, jump it back to a low squat position and rise to catch the ball. Your partner controls the toss and speed of the ball while you are executing the movements. Not only are you working your quads, glutes, pectorals and triceps, but this is an aerobic exercise guaranteed to liberate the endorphins.

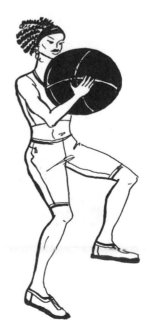

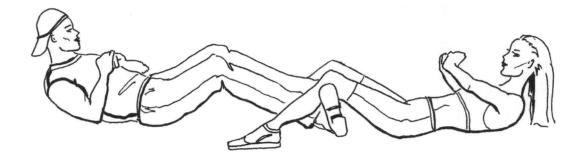

SIT-UPS IN TANDEM

Find a partner, sit on the ground, bend your knees and interlock your legs to transform an ordinary sit-up to a playful exercise. Come up together and come down together just to the shoulders' lifted position. Make sure to hold in your abdominals tightly and to exhale as you come up. When this becomes easy, if you wish to add intensity, you can throw a weighted medicine ball to one another when you lift up, as one of you takes it down. Do as many as you can. Aim for 3 sets of 15. If you don't have a partner, you can still have fun alone on the floor holding a medicine ball with bent knees doing this sit-up in front of a mirror!

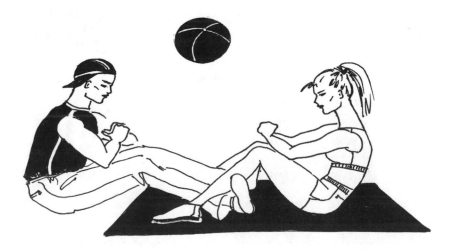

CHAPTER 12

TRAINING FOR THE NONCONFORMIST

Two roads diverged in a wood, and I –
I took the one less traveled by,
And that has made all the difference
Robert Frost

Nonconformists pride themselves on being high spirited, creative and independent. To the external world they appear rebellious, questioning cherished traditions and rituals. Some nonconformists tend to be artistic-- viewing the world from an original perspective. They can't help but see the world differently. Sometimes nonconformists spring out of their own survival instincts. If family problems or secrets exist to make childhood an insecure, frightening, or lonely place, some children become nonconformists out of necessity.

SOMETIMES BEING A NONCONFORMIST IS CONFORMIST

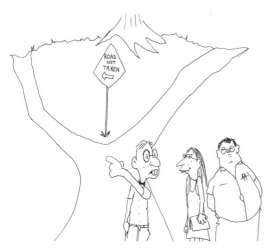

Because their family life does not fall into a "normal" category, they do not either. They become nonconformists to deal with their problematic or disturbing environments. Because they struggle from an early age, these children develop an inner strength, an inner need to question, "Why?" They learn to amuse themselves not with the traditional Ken and Barbie dolls or Lionel Train sets because they either never had them to play with in the first place, or subconsciously saw the mockery of their own existence reflected in these stereotypical idealized toys.

However, not every rebel is by definition a nonconformist. While it is the nature of teenagers to rebel and perceive adults as fools, actually, teenagers are conformists: they dress alike in their rebellion, and speak alike in their invented language. If one tries too hard to be a nonconformist, then he is obviously not a nonconformist. Sometimes people choose the road not taken for the sake of being different; it's chic or cool to be different. There can be great conformity in being a nonconformist. How difficult to walk the path of mediocrity and responsibility! Perhaps many choose the guise of the nonconformist because they are afraid that they will fail in school, on the job or in a relationship. Therefore, they don't even try; instead they do "their own thing."

When dealing with true nonconformists, one has to realize that the individual is generally a profound thinker who has a heightened awareness of social ills. Often that person wonders about his role in the universe. He is conscious of core relationships without regard to material wealth and diplomas. Cultivating his intuition and listening to it, the nonconformist trusts it more than the average person does. Therefore he will develop his artistic eye which is in fact his, original "I" voice, offering it to the world as a gift. If he is rejected and many times that is the case as Ralph Waldo Emerson said, "To be great is to be misunderstood," he is likely to get bored easily, or annoyed with superficialities. He does not hesitate to move away from others who are shallow and lack the profundity of thought or experience.

If you live with a nonconformist, or work with one, life can be exciting, but difficult. It is hard to reign in a nonconformist who might be compared to the maverick stallion on top of the hill. Also, since many are blunt or alienate themselves from the masses by virtue of their appearance or self-expression, they can be a bit rude. Then why do many nonconformists end up living with conformists? As the old saying goes, opposites attract. Also, these artistic types need an anchor when they become too quirky as they tend to get locked into a role of always being different. Did you ever notice that the children of nonconformists tend to be conservative, seeking structure and tradition?

Exercises for the nonconformist have to be constantly changing and unorthodox. Since the nonconformist tends to get bored, he needs constant stimulation. If the smith machine in the gym is used to train the pectoral muscles, he would delight in using it as a vertical leg press. Nonconformists need to vary their training exercises every few weeks. Also, explosive movements are popular with nonconformists, especially those incorporating both arms and legs, and quick reaction time.

If you wish to be less of a conformist in order to achieve balance in your personality, risk experiencing new things. Try to be spontaneous in your responses or actions. Tell people how you really feel. Be less accommodating to them, less diplomatic because the conformist in you needs to be well-liked by others. You can't go around being what everyone wants you to be and believe that you will be happy. Like an artist, you can create the world that you live in because it is internal. Take classes and read books in different subjects to explore and fulfill secret dreams and longings.

However, if you are a nonconformist who has surpassed nonconformity and wish to be more of a conformist in order to coexist, then try being more agreeable. Do a favor for a friend, even if you feel reluctant to interrupt your day. Go to your house of worship and sit in a pew with members of your community. Listen to other people, instead of issuing statements.

MIND/BODY PRESCRIPTIONS:

FOR THOSE WHO ARE TIRED OF CONFORMING
- Change your accustomed seat at the kitchen table.
- Wear an unusual hat.
- Don't match your clothes; wear something discordant.
- Get a children's coloring book and color outside the lines.
- Say this affirmation: "I am an original. I answer to myself and to no one else."

FOR THOSE WHO HAVE SURPASSED NONCONFORMITY
- Dress in conservative garb.
- Say "I see," instead of saying, "I disagree."
- Play a team sport.
- Buy a coloring book and color in the lines.
- Say this affirmation: "We are all part of a universal gate. We inhale and exhale each other."

MEDITATION:

A **meditation** for a nonconformist was not written because a nonconformist would not follow someone else's meditation.

MEDITATION TO HELP SHED CONFORMITY AND INVOKE ORIGINAL THINKING:
Sit with palms facing up. Close your eyes. Relax your breaths. Inhale and exhale to your own rhythm. Picture yourself on a white sandy beach. The sky is pale blue with tall green palm trees breaking through the horizon. Deep blue, turquoise waves rise and fall. Do you like this picture? Are you comfortable in this traditional setting? Bring your attention to your breathing. Are your breaths shallow or deep? Begin to breathe more deeply, inhaling and exhaling. Now erase these colors and repaint your landscape. Let your feelings color your picture. Have the colors changed? Is your sand green? Maybe the ocean is pink. Repaint the sky. Feel free to rearrange the scenery in your painting. You can move the trees, walk on water, or make the sand bloom. Take a moment to recreate the picture. Feel your impressions as you project yourself onto this new terrain. You create your thoughts and your thoughts create your new reality. Perhaps next time you will change it again. When you are ready, return to your surroundings. Open your eyes to see your world afresh. Now really open your eyes…Conform without conforming.

EXERCISES FOR THE NONCONFORMIST:

OBJECTIVE: TO STIMULATE ORIGINALITY WITH COMPOUND OR MULTI-JOINT EXERCISES

CHALLENGING HIKE

Take a challenging hike. Try to vary the terrain and the landscape. For an advanced workout add a weighted vest, or strap on a heavy backpack. Push yourself hard, but follow safety guidelines such as proper foot wear, adequate water, etc. Build up your stamina gradually.

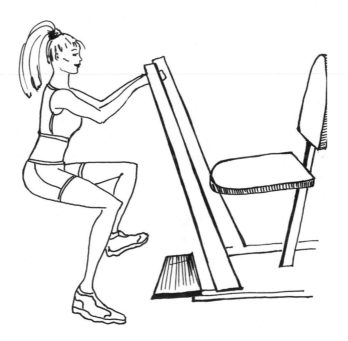

BACK ROW IN A CHEST PRESS MACHINE

*Transform a seated chest press machine at the gym into a back row. **Note:** This is an advanced movement. Squat in front of the chest press machine at arm's distance. Pull the handles with your arms bent just past 90 degrees toward your midsection. As you pull, concentrate on using your back muscles rather than your biceps. Visualize a quarter in your mid-back that you are squeezing together. Not only are you working your back muscles, but you are also working quadriceps and glutes. Adjust the weight according to ability. Aim for 3 sets of 10-12 repetitions.*

VERTICAL LEG PRESS

Transform a traditional smith machine used as a bench press into a vertical leg press. With legs shoulder distance apart in a 90 degree angle lift and lower the bar toward your ribs. Do not lock out your knees.
Safety note*: Pay attention to back support positioning before executing this movement. Do not lift your lower back which should be firmly planted. You can begin to add plates on the side in slow increments as this becomes easy. Begin with 3 sets of 10-12, gradually increasing to 3 sets of 25.*

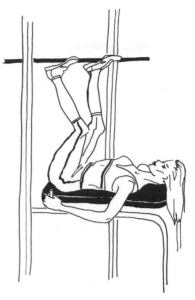

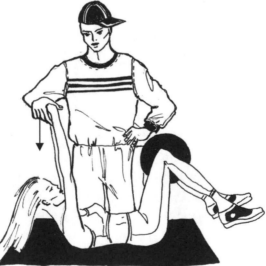

ABDOMINALS

*Try this abdominal exercise if you crave the unusual. Remember to hold your abdominals in tightly and to exhale as you rise. Hold a light ball between your thighs and lift your shoulders up as you push your back into the floor. Squeeze the ball between your legs at the same time. Return to the floor, but keep your shoulders raised. Then for the **next level** of intensity lift your shoulders as you crunch up and at the same time curl your legs toward you as you squeeze the ball. Try to lift off the tail bone-slightly when you curl your lower body, as this is a small move. For the most **advanced level**, you need a partner who will add some resistance to your arms which are extended up while you crunch upper and lower body squeezing the ball. Do as many as you can for each level of intensity. Aim for 25. Note that you are working inner thighs as well as abdominals.*

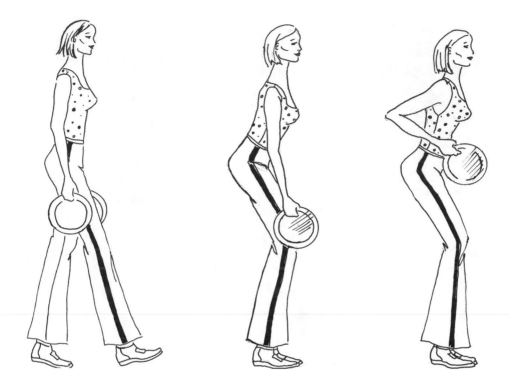

SQUAT BACK ROW

*For a **different** back exercise, carry two 10 lb plates and walk 8 steps. Then in a squat back row position, weight on the heels without arching the back, hold for 4 counts. Next pull the discs toward your back concentrating on squeezing your shoulder blades together as though you had a quarter you were squeezing in the middle of your back. Do 8 repetitions. Then stand up straight pushing off your heels and walk 8 steps. Repeat back and forth across a room—the bigger the room the better. This adds an aerobic component because you are walking while carrying weights as well as muscle training.*

CHAPTER 13

TRAINING FOR TECHNOLOGY

Come forth into the light of things,
Let nature be your teacher
William Wordsworth

Many of us long for the good old days, a simpler, more innocent, more gracious time. Memory provides a rose colored lens to view the past: once upon a time… Memory makes the tree we climbed when we were young grow taller, mom's cooking a lot tastier and our trudge to school a lot longer. However, we should be careful for what we wish when it comes to reliving the past as if our wishes could be granted anyway. Technology, its miracles and its horrors, is here to stay enmeshed with our lives. Progress appears to give us greater control like the precise hands of robotic heart surgery; however, if there is a malfunction, then the small chest incision made for the robotic hand gives the surgeon's hand far less control. Remember the dread of Y2K when computers could have brought our world to a grinding global halt, affecting: electricity, travel, water, surgery and banking. We would have lost control.

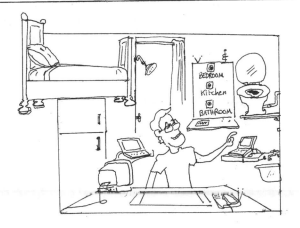

YOU NEVER HAVE TO LEAVE YOUR OFFICE

When technology overwhelms you, what do you do? You're on line five or six hours a day. You consult your palm pilot. Your car has a navigation system. You find yourself staring at screens, e-mailing key words, rather than speaking on the phone or writing letters. You can listen to music or view movies at your desk rather than go out; you can shop on line rather than select and touch the merchandise in stores. You can even have an affair on line without leaving home. You trade on the stock market and do all banking by computer. In short, you are addicted to the screen. Every few years you update your computer to have more memory, to function at a greater speed as it takes up less space. There is absolutely no need to leave your desk, which has become a microcosm.

Although the technological age has promised to free up more leisure time because of the swift calculations or the global distances computers integrate, we seem to be busier than ever before. We can be on line 24 hours a day if we wish. Leisure time is actually diminished.

Thus technology has brought the world to our fingertips, but its dark side has caused us to become more sedentary, lazier physically as the mind races along with the computer's brain. Therefore we lose our balance. Our minds are working on overdrive while our bodies are not exercising. A few extra pounds, even obesity, becomes a problem. We snack on fast foods while we stare at the screen, not paying attention to what we eat, or how quickly we consume it.

We need to go outdoors to cultivate our natural side. Taking a stroll or jogging restores our animal natures. We smell the air, feel the earth, see the sky and listen to the songs of birds. Even short walks indoors away from the computer provide us with a necessary respite. Looking out of a window into the horizon stretches our vision.

When we sit at our desk for too long, we tend to sit with poor posture. Very few of us sit with a straight back. Therefore we might feel pain in the lower back, or experience a pinched nerve in a cervical disc. If we sit with our legs crossed for too long, we put pressure on the blood vessels possibly causing varicose veins. Also, a common byproduct of long hours of typing on a keyboard is Carpal Tunnel Syndrome.

Stretching to release tension and stiffness gives the body a necessary break from its sedentary position. Elongating the body with an overhead stretch or a palm press relieves neck, shoulder and upper back tension. Then doing a torso stretch and a side stretch relieves hip and lower back tension. Spreading our fingers or pulling them apart relieves cramps. We feel relaxed and refreshed. We can then return to the computer and begin the cycle again.

Creating *natural* time and space stimulates our minds and bodies. We need to divest from unnecessary tasks in order to exercise, dance, play a sport, or do yoga. If our schedules don't permit, then we must change our schedules. When we refresh our bodies, they fuel our minds to work more creatively and efficiently. We cannot in the long run ignore the body's demands. When we are whole, our work is whole and of a better quality. In turn, our confidence is boosted, affecting business and familial relationships positively because of a well-rounded lifestyle.

MIND/BODY PRESCRIPTIONS:

- Turn off the screen. Eat lunch by yourself in an empty office or conference room. Create a corner of inner harmony without any distractions.
- On the way to and from work observe the beauty around you, a tree, an expressive face, the angle of the light.
- During work look out the window and see the cloud formations. Get back to nature; do not lose perspective of what is eternal.

MEDITATION:

DURING A COFFEE OR LUNCH BREAK

Sit comfortably with palms facing up. Begin your breathing practice. Close your eyes and imagine a day in the country. See yourself swinging in a knotted rope hammock connected to two tall hundred-year old oak trees. Swing slowly back and forth. Look up at the sky through green leaves and see the filtered dappled light. You feel warmed by the heat of the sun, yet are protected from its strong intense light by green oak leaves. Relax your body. Try to feel weightless as you swing in the hammock. Stretch out with your arms and feet spread wide apart on the net. Open and spread your fingers and toes. How does it feel to stretch out from one end of your body to the other? How does your mind feel? As you stretch and swing, back and forth, let your mind roam freely to settle on a natural scene. Expand what you see to a larger vista. Be there for another moment. Gradually transfer this image to your work station. Be mindful of your breaths. Begin to return to your computer screen; your body as well as your mind feels refreshed. When you are ready, open your eyes. You feel as though you have been away on a vacation and return alert, eager to handle your workload.

EXERCISES TO TRAIN FOR TECHNOLOGY:

OBJECTIVE: REBOOT YOUR SYSTEM

Walk to work. If that is impractical, then park your car and walk part of the way, or get off the train or bus one stop earlier. Climb the stairs to your office instead of taking the elevator. If you work on a very high floor, get off the elevator a few floors earlier and climb some stairs. Take a walk during your lunch break.

For those who want to break up their workday with a workout, check out a local gym during your lunch hour. If that's not a viable alternative, bring a pair of sneakers and a jump rope to work. 15 minutes of jumping rope (this does not have to be done consecutively; you can do short bursts of 2-3 minutes throughout the day) will provide a great aerobic workout, particularly effective for strengthening quadriceps and hamstrings. The explosive jumping movements burn many calories and prevent osteoporosis. And if you are frustrated and annoyed at work, you can whip your secretary with a jump rope or hang your boss! (Only kidding!)

Sitting at your desk for hours can make you stiffen. Take a break and move around. Look out the window to stretch your eyes which have been doing closely detailed work. The following are suggested stretches for your body. Hold each stretch for 15-20 seconds and breathe.

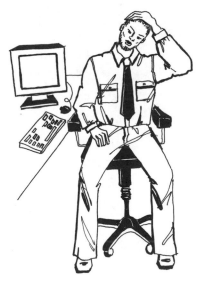

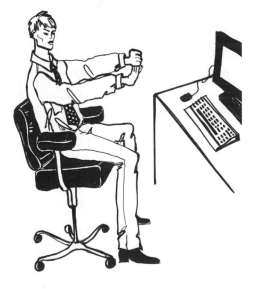

TARGETS NECK MUSCLES
Place one hand at the side of your head and gently push your head toward your shoulder. Return to the starting position. Repeat on the other side.

TARGETS FOREARM EXTENSION
Extend your arms in front of you and gently press your right hand against the top of your left fingers with your palm facing away from your body. Gently pull towards the body. Repeat on the other side.

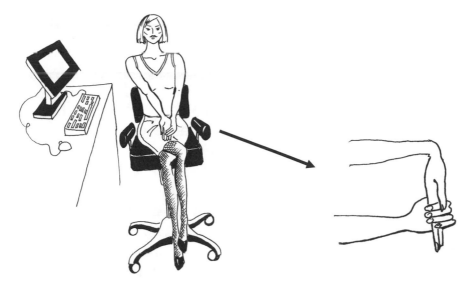

TARGETS FOREARM FLEXORS

Extend your left arm with your fingers pointing down, your palm facing away from your body. Apply gentle pressure with the right hand. Repeat on the other side.

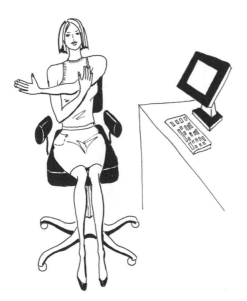

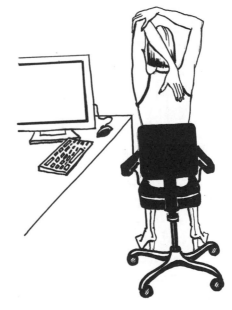

TARGETS SHOULDER RANGE OF MOTION

Extend your left arm across your chest. Apply gentle pressure with your right arm. Be sure not to press against your elbow joint. Repeat on the other side.

TARGETS TRICEPS

Raise your left arm and bend down with fingers touching mid-back. Take your right arm and gently apply pressure to keep the left arm down. Repeat on the other side.

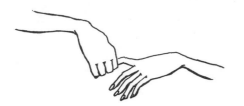

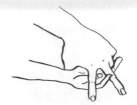

TO LOOSEN FINGERS AND PROMOTE DEXTERITY

Spread two fingers at a time and insert two fingers from your other hand and gently pull them apart—creating a V within a V. Repeat for all pairs of fingers on both hands.

TO LOOSEN FINGER JOINTS

Grasp each finger with the other hand and one at a time, gently pull.

WRIST FLEXIBILITY (Not Shown)

Rotate your wrists in the air with the fingers on your right hand moving clockwise and the fingers on your left hand moving counter clockwise. Then reverse direction.

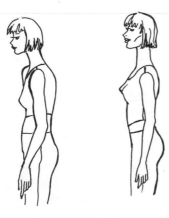

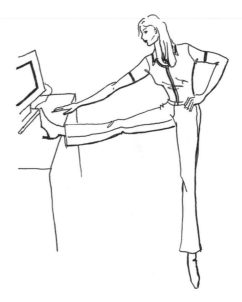

TARGETS OVERALL POSTURE AND SPINAL ALIGNMENT

Grounded in the earth, aspiring to the top - see what a difference posture makes. Stand tall and straight in the yoga Mountain Pose. Stand erect; feet together big toes touching, hips in a pelvic tilt, abdominals pulled into the back, squeeze the glutes so that the thighs are engaged. Shoulders drift down your back, chest is open, chin slightly tucked, crown of the head is pointed up aspiring toward the top. Your arms are at your sides, fingers pointing to the earth. Close your eyes as you actively remain still. Hold for 5 deep breaths.

TARGETS LOWER BACK AND HAMSTRINGS

Lift your leg and extend it out on your desk, or any table while maintaining your balance on the other leg. Gently, don't force it; reach toward your toes. Repeat on the other side.

CHAPTER 14

TRAINING FOR THE ADDICTIVE PERSONALITY

I do not know why this confronts me,
This sadness, this echo of pain;
A curious legend still haunts me,
Still haunts and obsesses my brain
Heinrich Heine

The colloquial expression that sums up the essence of addiction is: "too much of a good thing." Addictions and obsessions cover a wide range of objects: alcohol, drugs, smoking, gambling, sex, shopping, coffee, eating, not-eating, exercising, negative thoughts and of course, my personal favorite, chocolate. Some of us are born with a genetic predisposition to addiction. However, others acquire the habit through constant exposure or interaction with a specific combination of environmental factors. The rhetorical question arises if something makes me feel this good initially, what is wrong with wanting more? Who has not looked with glazed eyes, laughing that wicked laugh approaching the addiction source to swoop down on the prey? All of us are addicted to something or someone at some point in our lives. In fact, highly successful people obsess about work or a creative idea. They claim to be "driven." Many of us obsess about a new love object, devoting all our thoughts and energies to the other person. However, we have to distinguish romantic dreams from the dark side of daydreaming which disrupts inner peace. While addiction to success appears desirable, when it interferes with personal happiness creating an imbalance in our spiritual and physical makeup, then we must track it to the source. In other words, does being a workaholic stem from a fundamental feeling of worthlessness? Do we have to constantly prove ourselves?

Addiction is a sensory experience which sends pleasure signals to the brain. We rely on the transitory comfort addiction serves. The key word is transitory, for soon we need another high, or a higher dosage to achieve the same euphoria, as any shop-aholic will confess. Addiction, which usually connotes a loss of self-control, ironically, gives us a false sense of control, or empowerment. For example, when a person chooses not to eat, he believes that he has control over his body. When a person gambles, he tries to control his luck. When a person obsesses about a lover, he tries to control that lover.

When we become addicted, it is because deep down we believe that we have lost our power, or do not know how to tap into it. Therefore we find a stimulant to give us a sense of empowerment, or a substance to numb us. We become unnatural, out of balance, looking for distractions to avoid answering basic internal questions such as, "Why am I not happy?" The external distractions give us that temporary high—false happiness, an escape from the real problem.

Why do some teenage girls have a proclivity to anorexia, an addiction to not eating? Here is a possible theory. Their bodies are running hormonally rampant. They feel like women, yet still take orders from their parents. They are unsure about how to behave sexually, or are insecure and frightened by their sexuality. Often a boyfriend wields a controlling statement, "If you love me, you would do it." They feel powerless and out of balance. Therefore when they choose not to eat and see the tangible result of losing weight, teenage girls feel in control of their own bodies. In addition, they become "unfeminine in their thinness" looking more like a *petite gamine*, or a boy. They stop menstruating. They become asexual to avoid dealing with their ambivalence regarding sex.

The flip side of anorexia, overeating, is an addiction to food as comfort. We need to fill up because we are lacking fulfillment in our lives. What we are lacking is the perception that we are loved and will not be abandoned. We eat to give ourselves pleasure and comfort because our own spirit does not nurture us.

Similarly, the sex addict and the love addict need a constant flow of another person's energy to fill up what is lacking in his own personality. He drains the other person like a vampire because he is insecure and needs validation. He needs constant attention to recharge his energy because he fears his own company the most-- having never learned to be alone with the self. Also, the love addict has not taken responsibility for his personal happiness drawing it from others as he gives little in return. We have all been love addicts at one time or another, especially during the teenage years when we explored our identities. Remember the time when you had a crush on someone. You needed to get just a little peek or sneak in a little conversation to fuel the obsession. Sometimes you gave little gifts to the crush, or perhaps you went a bit overboard and stalked the object of your desire. Inevitably, most adult romances begin with compulsive thoughts in the form of hopes and dreams about the new date along with a need for a regular flow of compliments and promises. Eventually, when a relationship becomes established, routine settles in and the neediness dissipates. However, when this pattern continues to repeat itself for months, then most likely addiction holds an insecure person in a vise grip.

Addictions, mild or serious, point to our need for self-completion. Some of us who are strong willed and intuitive about our ailments can heal by going cold turkey, throwing away that last cigarette. Some of us need to bottom out, confronting the reality of the abyss before we can transform ourselves into a self-loving individual. Most of us who are addicted need professional help or *Twelve Step Programs* with group support to free ourselves from physical and mental slavery. Since others who have experienced the same addiction share their stories and power resources, a circle of wisdom is created to circulate good energy and spirituality.

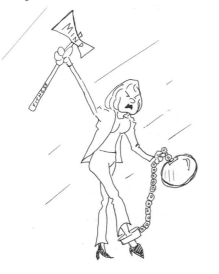

While gyms are replete with people seeking fitness, health and a better life quality, exercise addicts can be found in every gym. These women and men stay in the gym for hours, abusing mind and body. They take two or three classes back to back and then get on a treadmill or a stair climber to do more. Many lift weights for over two hours a day, overtraining, sometimes causing bodily injury. Rather than starve or vomit, these exercisers eat, but then work off what they ate and then some! Like other addicts, they feel insecure and powerless. Therefore working out all day provides the illusion of control over muscles. Because they feel unfulfilled and unhappy, they work out for hours at a time to get their endorphins up, with the increasing need for more exercise to maintain happy feelings and personal empowerment.

Sometimes people are addicted to more than one thing concurrently, for example: smoking, sex, shopping, gambling, or exercise. Even when addictive people proclaim their freedom from a particular addiction, they tend to exchange it for another.

Addictive personalities are starved for validation. A good beginning for the emerging addict is to express these specific concerns and fears openly. He needs to embrace body and spirit, content to be alone and still. While relationships are necessary mirrors, the addict needs to establish and respect boundaries in these relationships. Otherwise these relationships become addictive as well. *He needs to expand his own world without contracting or draining another's.* Addicts are looking for others to complete them. However, no one can complete the self, but the self. While a relationship can be healing, it cannot be a substitute for the important work one must do alone.

One of the hardest things to accept when we are addicted is living in *ambiguity.* Because there are no absolutes in life, we tend to feel insecure. We need to come to terms with ambiguities: love, friendship, success and self-image. We accept that we will never truly, absolutely know for sure, because how do we quantify abstractions like love or self-esteem? When we realize that we are powerful beyond measure, we no longer need concrete validation; we can shed the addiction. Deep down we all know to be unequivocally true that each one of us has a bright light to offer the world. When someone challenges you, "Who are you to consider yourself to be brilliant?" A suggested response: "Who am I not?"

MIND/BODY PRESCRIPTIONS: 👁

CHANGE YOUR ROUTINES AND RITUALS

- Begin by changing your underwear (under ware). Wear a new color that you have never worn before. Perhaps it is the color, yellow, which symbolizes intellectual energy. For it is through your intellect that you will control your addiction.
- Break the pattern: wear your underwear inside out. Confront your addiction by bringing awareness to it
- Clean out your drawers. Organize your possessions. Get rid of what you don't need.
- Take hot showers, or go to a sauna to release toxins through the skin.
- Eat plenty of fiber; drink water and juice to clean out the toxins lodged in the body.
- Envision yourself healthy and happy because you have released the physical and/or emotional toxins in your life.

MEDITATION: 🧘

Sit up with dignity palms facing down. Look up towards your eyebrows and close your eyes. Be conscious of your breathing. Inhale and exhale. Try to inhale two counts, hold for one count and then exhale four counts—through the nose. Imagine a heavy iron shackle around your ankle. Look down at your leg iron. Touch it. Feel its weight. You see a word written on the collar. What word is it? Take a moment to decipher it. Observe yourself trudging around. Wherever you go, the iron shackle drags along. Let your body feel it. You wish you could be free and light. Continue to breathe, inhale and exhale. Now visualize a medieval skeleton key. You know that you own the key, but you have forgotten where you put it. Search your pockets and your bag, but still no key turns up. Try to focus on it in your mind's eye. Feel its texture. Take a deep breath and exhale completely. When you are ready, reach inside yourself and retrieve the key. See yourself unlock the shackle. Hear the sound of freedom. Experience it for a moment. You are free to move. Celebrate the lightness of being. See yourself moving forward and away. When you are ready, return to your surroundings. Open your eyes to living your true identity. You have brought peace to your higher and lower nature.

EXERCISES FOR THE ADDICTIVE PERSONALITY:

OBJECTIVE: NOT TO RUN AWAY FROM YOURSELF

To break an exercise addiction evidenced by more than 90 minutes of continuous exercise 7 days a week, the prescription calls for *no* exercise for one month. Overtraining causes feelings of depression and worthlessness. By resting the body, we heal the mind. Instead of being distracted, we face our inner demons that drive us to overload our muscles and connective tissues. We take the time to reflect on our restlessness and escapism. Where are we running to on a treadmill? Where do the stairs we are climbing lead? Are we getting nowhere fast as we pedal? Are we spinning out of control? When we can answer these questions, we can return to the gym. Meanwhile rest your muscles, enjoy your food and take the time to reevaluate goals and body image. During a resting phase muscles heal and grow. When you return to the gym, your muscles bounce back quickly because they retain "muscular memory." Here is the schedule: After the first week of inactivity, you may take a daily 30 minute walk (preferably outdoors) and see it as an opportunity to relax both mind and body. After 2 weeks you may ride a bike in the neighborhood. Within a month you can ease back into the gym, but with a prescribed time limit. If you have taken a month off from your workouts, surely you can take a week off every 6-8 week cycle?

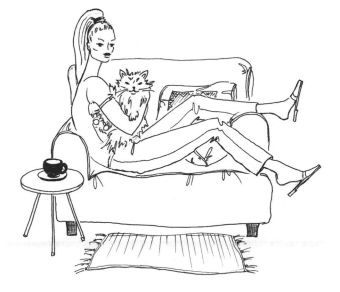

REST
Hold any position you like
for as long as you like.

CHAPTER 15

TRAINING FOR DECEPTION

The easiest person to deceive is one's own self
Edward Bulwer Lytton

We are born trusting the adults who give us life, take care of us and teach us. We elevate them on pedestals. We grow up filled with stories: fairytales, fables, myths, legends and parables. The good people are always rewarded and live happily ever after while the bad people are not only punished; their punishments fit the crime. Our eyes open wide as we begin to see the inconsistencies, the contradictions in the real world. We realize that the fairytale world is a deception. However, this statement needs to be qualified. If we re-read fairytales with experienced eyes, we realize that the deception is there for us to recognize. Fairytales are meant to reveal the deceptive characters that people our lives. For example, a wolf in proverbial sheep's clothing lures the unsuspecting sheep to follow him. A wolf disguised as Little Red Riding Hood's grandmother tries to devour the girl. A gingerbread house is used as a lure to trap innocent children like Hansel and Gretel. A queen disguises herself as an old woman handing Snow White a poison apple in the osten-

sible gift of friendship. Zeus assumes many shapes like a giant swan, golden rain, or a bull to seduce and impregnate the women he desires without his wife Hera knowing about it. From an early age we learn that deception slithers into our lives often catching us unaware like the serpent in Eden.

We have to be alert to spot deception and protect ourselves from the physical and mental pain it causes. Essentially there are two kinds of deception. The deception others practice and self-deception.

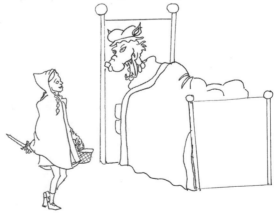

YOU CAN CHANGE THE STORY

Often we are deceived because we are lazy. We want to believe the lie, the easy smile, the sweet complimentary words that easily trip off the tongue. In order to see truth we have to work hard to study a person's eyes, body language, or tone of voice. We note if that person is making eye contact or looks away. When we concentrate on the words, are there any inconsistencies? Some promises cannot be delivered even if movie stars or superheroes say the words with conviction; as the old saying goes, if it is too good to be true, then it usually isn't. For example, an easy fix to weight loss is promised on TV or in magazines-- exercise in a bottle. Some of these bottles have proven worthless or even harmful! The truth is simpler and more mundane: calories in and calories out. If your caloric intake is greater than your caloric output, after taking exercise into consideration, then you will gain weight, not lose it! How much easier it is to believe the story!

At other times we are deceived not by another person, but by ourselves. Because we grew up on a diet of fairytales and legends, we love to represent things as we wish them to be. Therefore we hear what we want to hear and believe what we need to believe to fulfill hopes and dreams. We wear rose colored glasses distorting reality. We believe the contractor who consistently does not show up to work, or does shoddy carpentry when he promises that he will finish the job beautifully and on time! We believe that if we buy all the anti-aging cosmetics on the market, we will look as young as we did when we were in our twenties. We believe the, "I love you," said in the backseat of a car is not meant to seduce, but is a mystical confession of love.

The following scenario exemplifies the fairy tale world we tend to recreate in our lives. A woman found a dying snake in her backyard garden. She carried it into her house placing him in a basket near her warm hearth. She fed him mice and gave him the medicine that she purchased in a pet store. In short, she nursed him back to health. One day surprisingly the snake lurched forward and bit her on the hand without any provocation. The woman felt hurt. She asked the snake why he bit her after she had fed him and sheltered him for a month. The snake answered, "Because I am wild and it is my nature. What did you expect from a snake?" She had deceived herself into believing that she had changed his nature.

The time has come to remove your rose colored glasses and see the world's true colors which are rich and beautiful. Rather than providing a favorable tint, your rose colored glasses actually obscure the distinct depth and range of the color spectrum. Find a true friend with whom you can be sincere and who will be sincere with you. Share perceptions and ask that friend's opinion about your view of things. Does your friend see a pattern in your self-deception that you don't? Then progress to the next step. Try to befriend yourself. Don't act as your own enemy in deceiving yourself.

Think about why you want to be deceived. Is it because you are lonely and looking for love? Do you feel unattractive? Do you feel insignificant? Unrecognized or rewarded for your true potential? Instead of creating a false story to satisfy your needs or feed your insecurities, work on the real you. The following process will help you to change your perception about yourself. Begin by writing your childhood story as you have always interpreted it. For example: the little girl whose father did not love her; the little boy who was never good enough or smart enough; the child who felt lonely and abandoned. Next read your story aloud to yourself five times a day for a week. Then call up a close friend and have him or her do likewise. Read your stories to each other five times a day for a week. At this point you will be thoroughly nauseated by your story. Almost miraculously you will let it go and be free. You will rewrite your future by giving up your interpretation of the past. Perhaps, your interpretation was false in the first place, clean from the purpose of what really happened.

Proceed to clean out your closet throwing out all the outlandish equipment you bought impulsively to trim your thighs, abdomen, and butt. Throw out the rollers, the crunchers, and the vise grips. Call a meeting with a group of sincere friends and ask them if you need to lose any weight. If they feel that you do, start a legitimate weight loss and exercise program. There are no short cuts. Transform your body realistically through diet and consistent exercise.

Then go to your medicine cabinet and throw out the anti-wrinkle creams, cellulite reduction creams, fountain of youth creams and anti-aging lotions. Hearing them smash in the garbage can provides an added satisfaction. Do purchase and use a sun block with an SPF of 15 or higher to protect and conserve your skin. Avoid intense sun, keep your face clean and use a moisturizer. Smile a lot. You will look years younger.

In order to heighten your awareness of deception, learn about body language, tone of voice and verbal cues. As the saying goes, knowledge is power. Knowledge will provide you with the self-confidence to critically evaluate what is real and what is a façade. Look at credentials and qualifications. Observe and discern if they are truly deserved. Learn to cultivate your inner radar, your intuition, to distinguish between appearance and reality. Use your inner focus when you weight train. The more you "dig in" by using your third eye to hold the weight in a static contraction or complete the extra repetitions beyond the burn, the more you will develop a sixth sense. When you have done thirty squats with a weighted bar on your upper back and your legs begin to hurt because of the buildup of lactic acid, do five more. Say to your self, "There is nothing I can't accomplish. I know I have more in me." What you are actually doing is forecasting your success. You are concretely demonstrating your ability to see further down the road with your third eye. Once you have learned to draw from your inner focus during your workouts and trust its ability, you will naturally do the same in daily life. Deception will slither away, defeated, unable to infiltrate or transform your goodness into cynicism.

MIND/BODY PRESCRIPTIONS:

DISPEL DECEPTION

◆ Don't believe the myth of spot training. "I can do fifteen minutes of sit-ups daily to reduce the fat deposits around my middle." In truth sit-ups will help build strong abdominals, but those muscles will not be visible unless you do enough aerobics to lose the adipose tissue that covers them as well. Also remember that if you do not hold your abdominals in tightly as you do your sit-ups, pulling your naval into your back, you might just build those abdominals out.

◆ Don't believe the myth of working out for many hours at a time. "If one hour of aerobics is good, then three or four is better." However, the body adjusts to this intense workout, and now you end up having to do five or six hours to effect a change for the better. The law of diminishing returns kicks in. Better to cross train, mix aerobics with weight training to make a change and don't go beyond ninety minutes. More is less.

◆ Do learn about correct form. Then you will know enough to avoid a trainer or instructor who is *not* qualified to work with you. Interview trainers and clients, or watch a training video to gain enough knowledge to spot a charlatan. Just because someone looks buffed does not mean he can teach. Appearances can be deceiving.

◆ Hold a position long enough to recruit your third eye. For instance, do planks for the lower body, or push-ups for the upper body; then hold that position.

◆ Do five more reps in weight training from the point where you "think" you can go no further.

◆ Study fairy tales and myths with adult eyes. Analyze their psychology and social commentaries.

◆ Recall a favorite fairytale. See which character resembles you and why.

◆ Notice the distinct aromas in your environment. What emotion or memory does each smell evoke? Cultivate your primal nature.

◆ Get in touch with your inner feelings. Record sensory experiences that come up for you when: someone says no, you are happy, you are afraid, etc. Write a list of your personal sensory symbols. For example, when I am happy I smell cookies baking in the oven. Then when a situation arises and you smell cookies in the oven, you can determine that the situation is positive based on your own intuition.

◆ Intuition is natural and everyone possesses it in varying degrees. The good news is that the more you cultivate it, the more it grows. Even if you think you are not receiving any intuitive impressions, make something up. Surprisingly, in your fictional story lies your inner truth.

MEDITATION:

Sit with dignity, palms facing upward. Close your eyes and begin your breathing practice. Recall the story of "Little Red Riding Hood." Take a moment and become Little Red Riding Hood. While you are on your way to grandma's house, you meet the wolf. Visualize the scene as though the movie were playing on a screen in your head. See if you can change the script. Although your role is to be innocent and good, you are not naïve. You see through the deception. How do you feel about outsmarting the deceiver? Focus on the clue that awakened your intuition and put all your senses on high alert. Go into your body and feel the awareness for a moment. Your intuition lies in your solar plexus (located just below the navel), your gut feelings. Gradually open your eyes. Try to become aware of these primal feelings in your daily real life stories and begin to get in touch with your intuition. Read life.

EXERCISES TO SEE THROUGH DECEPTION:

OBJECTIVE: CORE TRAINING STRENGTHENS INNER KNOWING

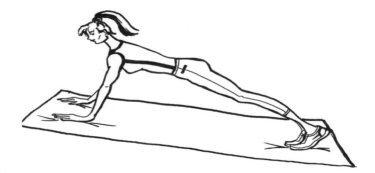

PUSH-UP POSITION

Get into push-up position and hold for 10 seconds. Make sure that you balance your body on your hands and toes, holding your abdominals in tightly. Keep your glutes lowered to form a straight line with your back. As you progress, increase your holding time in gradual increments of 10 seconds up to a minute. **Note:** *the strength for this position comes from your center, not your hands. Recruit your core muscles for support. For the most advanced move you can have a partner place a 10 lb plate on your upper back for 10 seconds gradually increasing to 30 seconds. Then after having maintained a holding position for a few weeks and that becomes easy, try a 25 pound disc on your upper back. Recruit the focus of your third eye to keep you steady.* **Remember to breathe and hold your abdominals in tightly.**

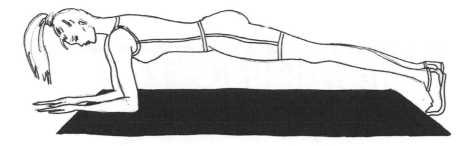

THE PLANK

Get down on the floor on all fours; then bend your elbows and place your palms flatly on the ground. Lift up off your toes, keeping your body in a straight line as you **hold your abdominals in tightly***. Maintain this position for 10 seconds, gradually increasing to 30 seconds and then to a minute. As you advance, for greater intensity, lift and lower your body from the waist down only, gently touching the floor. This is a lower body push-up. Tighten your glutes and hamstrings as you lift, lower and hold to maximize this exercise. Do 3-5 lower body push-ups for 3 sets and then hold for 10 seconds in plank position. In the last set after 3 lower body push-ups, hold for 10 seconds and then do 3 additional lower body push-ups. This breaks momentum. Increase the repetitions as you get stronger to 10 lower body push-ups per set and a 30 second plank hold to break momentum in the middle of each set. This exercise strengthens your "gut" feeling and your back, so that you will be able to "watch your back."*

ABDOMINALS PILATES STYLE

Lie on your back with your legs forming a 90 degree angle. Hold your abdominals in tightly as you press your lower back into the floor. Lift off the shoulders and press your arms down a couple of inches towards the floor. Press your arms down for 10 repetitions for 3 sets, gradually increasing to 25 repetitions per set. Tip: Pump your arms slowly and with control. Concentrate on pushing your arms down to the pull of gravity.

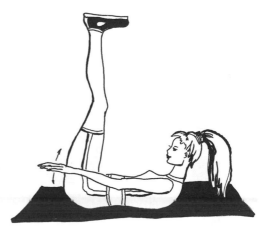

CHAPTER 16

TRAINING TO BE PATIENT

Adopt the pace of nature; her secret is patience
Ralph Waldo Emerson

One of the hardest traits to cultivate in life is patience. The child in us wants our needs attended to *immediately*. What distinguishes a spoiled child is his need for instant gratification, while a calmer, more behaved child accepts the answer, "later, we'll look forward to it." If we want to lose weight or get into shape, many of us need to see results the next day. If we learn a new sport like golf or tennis, we want to excel immediately, after our first lesson. If we order furniture, we want it the next day.

However, with negative emotions like grief, hurt, anger and despair, our impatience to get over each condition rises to a high point. When we experience pain, we become impatient. We become confused about how to deal with the source. All we can think of is living pain-free. But the universe has sent us pain to relay a specific message. To be alive is to feel pain. If we feel grief because someone has died, we have to release the old feelings in order to receive the new. Psychologists always remind us never to cut the grieving process short. If we rush through it, our sadness will drown us at a later date. If we are angry, then we grow impatient with the person who has triggered this response. But in essence, we need to discover why we have empowered this person to make us angry. This discovery takes time. If we rush the internal investigation, we will repress the true source of our anger, triggering a variety of physical ailments, even a depressed immune system.

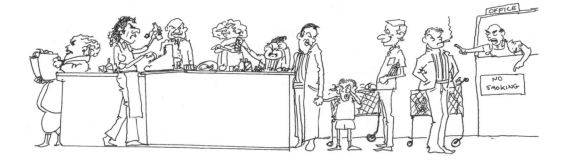

When we grow pessimistic about our goals or relationships, we are experiencing a stage in life where we need to gradually let go of established patterns, to be prepared for exciting transformations. We tend to be impatient with the process when we are letting go. As the saying goes, "old habits die hard." Therefore we have to be reasonable about expectations and be more patient. If we rush the process of discerning a pattern, we might not be able to see our role in the process, "It's not my fault," which means that we will most likely repeat the same disappointing pattern. For example, the first time I drive into a pothole on a certain street, it's an accident. The second time, I have to accept responsibility. The third time I realize there is another possibility-- go around the pothole. Ultimately, the goal is to drive up another street.

Learning patience slows us down and helps us consciously experience life instead of running in different directions, filled with distractions. Let us be like a windmill. *A windmill waits for the wind.* Being patient with others, we practice tolerance and forgiveness as we learn to be patient with ourselves. When someone lashes out at us, anger can be dissipated by calm, patient listening, instead of confronting the storm head on with hasty angry words that escalate the argument. A willow that can patiently bend during a hurricane waiting for the storm to pass is less likely to be uprooted.

When we are patient with ourselves, we lighten the tense burden of accomplishment. We need not compete with others, their riches or their status. When we don't feel impatient about our goals adhering to stressful timetables, we can enjoy the process. Why do we strive for perfection and does it even exist? We can stumble, or even fail, taking the time to learn from our failure to continue to the next success. When we rest and collect our thoughts, we get in touch with our internal energy. Just as our muscles grow during periods of rest following intense exercise, so do our souls.

Time is in the mind. In order to cultivate patience, let us perceive time as subjective. What if we were on an island with no clocks or calendars? In fact, whenever we are involved in a hobby we love, we lose track of time. *Note: when we lose track of time, we do not age.* However, since we do have external clocks and calendars, we can still create internal, timeless moments to work on breathing techniques, making them deeper, slower and more deliberate: to be conscious of each breath from where it is coming and going. In addition, as a natural companion to relaxed breathing, we might try to set aside a time and place for meditation, or affirmative visualizations. Patiently, we wait for an image or a word to come to mind as a loving guide.

To be patient means to have the grace of acceptance as well as the opposing capacity for transformation because we are motivated and have a vision. Once we have slowly and me-thodically considered our feelings about our goals, we are ready to move on to the next level of consciousness towards achieving, or implementing. Likewise if we are not pleased with our bodies' health, fitness and appearance, then we can patiently change through exercise and diet. We will see improvement within one month. And this patient, gradual improvement will last far longer than any fad diet, fat-burning, or appetite suppressant pills and high tech cellulite massager that promise to melt away fat deposits. We will have changed our mindset to positively perceive fitness from the inside out, a healthy lifestyle. "Good things come to the one who waits."

Women, who have recently given birth, when the exhilaration of delivery is over, tend to complain about how their bodies look, impatient to lose the weight they put on during pregnancy. However, it took nine months to put on all that weight, shifting internal organs and stretching the skin. It seems logical that one must allow a few months to regain muscle tone, shed pounds, and increase skin elasticity. Often in the gym one can hear trainers telling new mothers, "Be patient. The weight will come off. Don't overdo." When women grow impatient, they sometimes give up, "What's the use? It'll never happen. I'll never look as good as I did before. I might as well give up exercising and eat to satisfy my frustration." However, I have observed that when women are patient with their bodies and believe in a healthy process, they not only achieve their pre-pregnancy state, but look even better than they ever did before!

MIND/BODY PRESCRIPTIONS:

SLOW DOWN AND BE METHODICAL

- Tai Chi incorporates slow, fluid movements, which can be performed well into old age. In fact, tai chi promotes longevity.
- Walk with 3-5 pound ankle weights to slow you down.
- When ordering furniture, an appliance, or an art work, insist on a delayed delivery.
- Purposely select an extremely slow serving restaurant when you feel hungry.
- Make a doctor's appointment and insist that everyone else precede you, "after you."
- Choose the slowest line in the supermarket and read a magazine while you wait.
- Sit in your car in heavy traffic listening to music or book tapes.
- Tutor someone in a subject of your specialty.
- Ask someone to teach you something that is difficult for you to learn, so that you can experience being on the receiving side of impatience.
- Do not wear your wrist watch for a day.
- Plant a seed and watch it grow.

MEDITATION:

Close your eyes as you sit with your palms facing up. Relax your breathing. Inhale and exhale mindfully. See yourself on top of a mountain. Experience the blue sky and white peak. Your vision is clear and you can see for miles without any obstruction. Inhale the cool brisk air allowing your body to feel invigorated. Find a huge rock to perch on. Is there a pressing question on your mind? Is there an issue in your life that needs immediate resolution? Take a few deep breaths of fresh oxygen. Know that by waiting and trusting, the universe will provide you with guidance. Bring your attention back to your breath. Allow your body to relax more as it releases its tension. Muscles and joints loosen as you begin to feel infinitely flexible. You lose all sense of time to experience a timeless awareness. There is only you and nature. You do not feel alone, rather a significant part of the grand scheme of things. Adopt the pace and freedom of nature. There are no deadlines and pressures. Whatever does not get done today will get done tomorrow. The sky darkens and is lit by stars and moonlight. You wait for guidance. The sky brightens with sunlight and white wispy clouds. You wait for guidance. You are not hungry, thirsty, or worried. You see an eagle flying overhead. Perhaps this image is your answer. Listen attentively. You hear the howl of a wolf in the distance. Perhaps this primal call is your answer. Wait for an image to come to mind. How do you feel about your urgent goals and needs? Carry this image back to your reality to help you patiently wait for enlightenment. Remember enlightenment can happen at any time when you are calm and not distracted. Be receptive to the answer. The process is creative, moving in its unhurried pace through time and space. Go beyond your thoughts and ideas about how things should be. Try to see things in a different light. Gradually, journey back to your original surroundings with feelings of contentment and calmness. Open your eyes to your own relaxed accomplishment.

EXERCISES TO BE PATIENT:

OBJECTIVE: TO MAINTAIN A VISION, ENJOY THE PROCESS AND REACH IT WITHOUT A TIME LIMIT

DEEP STRETCHING

Indulge in deep stretching with a partner. Breathe in and out as you keep your hip down, leg straight up, knee relaxed and foot flexed. Your partner will carefully and gently guide your leg toward you as you inhale and exhale. Over the course of time, experience how your leg moves closer to your shoulder as your partner gently guides it. Repeat for each leg holding for 20-30 seconds. Remember to relax and breathe deeply.

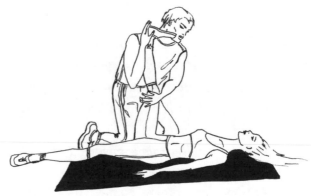

TOUCH YOUR TOES

In a seated position on the floor, first raise your arms straight up overhead and then lower and bend to reach your toes. Go as far as you can, without pain or force. Remember to inhale and exhale through your nose. Hold your stretch for 20-30 seconds. Repeat the whole sequence 3 times. Notice by the third time that you reach a little farther. After a few weeks, or months you will reach your toes.

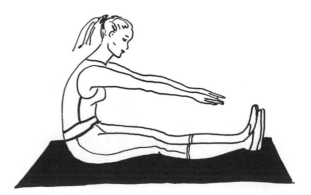

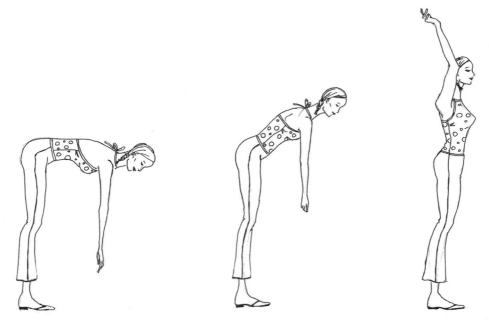

BACK STRETCH

Reach down toward your toes with your back straight to form an imaginary table. Hold your abdominals in tightly and keep your legs straight. Then patiently lift up one vertebra at a time, very slowly, breathing in and out through your nose. Imagine that your hands are a fountain dripping water. When you rise to your full height, extend your arms up, slightly behind your head. Repeat the entire sequence and this time when you lower, bend your knees as you touch the floor with the palms of your hands and then lift up to straighten your back and your legs to form a table with your arms dropping as far as they naturally go. Repeat your rise the same way as before. Do 3 repetitions.

PATIENT SUGGESTIONS

- ◆ *Take a spinning class for the first time. You will want to have the speed and strength that others demonstrate in class. You will learn about a resistance knob that **you control** to spin at your own pace. In the beginning set the resistance knob at a lower level than other participants. By the third class you can pedal with the resistance knob at a higher level. By the eighth or the tenth class you will become proficient and keep up with the instructor.*
- ◆ *The same applies to weights. You may want to lift heavier weights, or put more plates on each machine. Begin slowly when you add plates. Work with five to ten pound increments. Patience lets your body adjust to overload, building up muscle fiber gradually boosting strength and endurance. If you do not gradually increase weights, but overload the muscle suddenly, you risk permanent injury. After a few months of patient training, you will be lifting the weights you wanted to lift the first time you trained. Your initial visualization will have come true now that you are duly prepared*

CHAPTER 17

TRAINING TO YIELD

To go with the drift of things,
To yield with a grace to reality
And bow and accept the end
Of a love or a season?
Robert Frost

According to Zen philosophy we can overcome an obstacle by yielding; softness overcomes hardness. In Aikido, a form of martial arts, you never oppose an aggressor's strength head on. Instead, the idea is to yield to an oncoming force in such a way that it is unable to harm you, yet at the same time redirecting its strength away from you. Do not push or attack, but gently guide the force where you wish. This principle easily translates to problems that arise in daily life. Because each one of us has an ego and wants to be right, many confrontations can be deflected by letting other people be right, too. Don't meet a harangue head on. Listen quietly. Then deflect the harsh words by politely acknowledging the merit of the opposition's argument, while calmly interjecting your own point. Sometimes it helps to summarize your opponent's key points before adding your own: "If I understand you correctly…"

In our Western culture we have often heard the proverb, "God give me the grace to accept that which I cannot change." Because we are created in God's image, sometimes we tend to feel Godlike, or in other words in the driver's seat. People in our lives become pawns, or characters in our stories. We tend to see arguments or situations solely from a subjective perspective. We forcefully try to compel our friends, co-workers and lovers to do things our way and in our time frame. However, each one of us writes a different story and we all want to play the lead role. Consequently, we become pawns and characters in other people's stories. Conflict ensues, a battle of personal stories, a test of wills. We feel stressed, depleted and negative. Ultimately, if opponents are evenly matched, nothing gets accomplished.

However, when we yield, we demonstrate faith in the universe that God will provide. The universe will honor us if we have the right motives, especially those that create harmony for everyone concerned. We see ourselves as part of a larger plan allowing us to release the burden of the ego and its suspicions. When we release our dammed up tensions, our energy flows more freely from ourselves to others who in turn feel more at ease about trusting us.

What is most important is to allow our energy to flow rather than to become blocked by conflict, or a battle of wills. For when we insist on conquering, we intensify the opposing will of the person we sought to control. We create a counterproductive situation, at worst overtly hostile and at best passive-aggressive behavior by the other person who pretends to cooperate. Anyone with a teenager in the house knows that you cannot compel him with the force of your will. You cannot make him study or order him not to drink. He can easily sit in his room with his book open wide and upside down, not reading a word. He can promise not to drink, but do so anyway without your knowledge. Having faith in his integrity as well as his ability to learn from the consequences will strengthen his sense of right and wrong. Ultimately, it helps everyone concerned when you yield to his personal maturational timetable. Try to send him affirming thoughts and messages, both verbal and spiritual, instead of commands and accusations.

Many of us stiffen our necks over a business partner who is not working according to our schedule, while we feel that we shoulder all the responsibilities. However, we cannot compel our partner's creative juices or accomplishments to conform to our time-table, nor need we conform to his. All of us know that nagging accomplishes nothing, yet we do it anyway to vent our frustrations. We do not flow with positive energy. If we are honest, we will acknowledge the manipulation: Do we perceive our partner as working for us or with us? When we manipulate others, we show a lack of respect and we disturb their harmony. Instead we can give up control and let our partner schedule and implement the project. Once he is in charge, the roles will reverse, for we have surrendered our force, designed to attribute guilt.

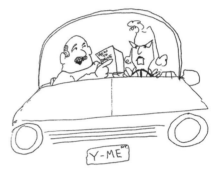

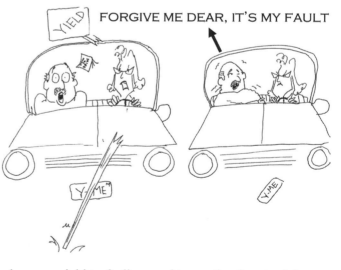

FORGIVE ME DEAR, IT'S MY FAULT

Yielding is a lot like love. We cannot compel another to love us, nor can we dissect love intellectually. In love we yield to feelings and to another heart, giving up control of our fortress to expose our vulnerabilities-- or else we will experience a diminished relationship. If we are not truly vulnerable in love, if we do not truly yield body and soul by opening up our feelings to our partners, then we lack the depth and sensuality that true love offers us. We can be safe and in control, but we can never be truly happy! In yielding lie ease, flexibility and great strength of spirit. When we yield to another, we are most secure in personal identity.

The utmost test of the human spirit is when we are ill. We know that in order to heal we need to actively partner our own healing with the medical community. While we do all the necessary things to get well for mind and body, we must also engage in the paradox of healing. We proactively take treatment as we yield to the disease. Like life-giving water, we collect ourselves and our energy to rise above the level of the illness, or else go around it in the same way that water will flow over or around a rock in its path. By yielding to sickness, we rest and restore to grow stronger. When we are sick and tired, we must take the time to find out what are we sick and tired of—emotionally and spiritually. Healing is holistic.

We know how to yield when we exercise. We yield to our bodies when they feel tired. We yield to instructors' and trainers' classes and programs. We perform the sequence of exercises, not knowing how many or what is next, but we trust the instructor. For many it seems more natural in a gym. Let it become more natural in our lives…

MIND/BODY PRESCRIPTIONS:

- ◆ Yield to a partner, a friend, a lover, or a relative in an argument where you are sure that you are absolutely right.
- ◆ Accept when a significant other says it is over, and believe it!
- ◆ Yield to your body; when you are tired, rest.
- ◆ Carry a small white flag with you. Use it often.

MEDITATION:

Sit with palms facing upward. Close your eyes. Relax your breaths. Inhale and exhale; become one with the universe. Imagine yourself riding a beautiful chestnut stallion in a green country-side. Feel the warm breeze caress your face. Inspire the natural fragrance of the meadow. The stallion directs the journey. Follow the winding path that brings you before an enormous castle. Notice the details of the architecture. How do you feel? The drawbridge is lowered. Allow yourself to dismount your horse. Fearful emotions may come up at this time. Don't judge them. Continue to breathe deeply. When you are ready, enter the castle. Instinctively, you remove your armor and lay down your sword. Return to your breath. Are you experiencing vulnerability? Whatever emotions you have, take them with you as you explore the surroundings. A scent of freshly prepared food wafts through the air. You sit down at a long mahogany table and eat heartily. Your eyelids grow heavy after the big meal and the long journey. Continue to relax your breath. You yield to your weariness and go to sleep in one of the many bedrooms. You wake up in a sunlit room, sensing that someone is in the castle with you. As you descend the stairs, your host greets you. A glimmer of recognition comes upon you. To whom have you really yielded your weapon and armor? How do you feel about yielding to him or her? Carry this breakthrough into your reality. Slowly return to your body. Open your eyes and smile at how good it feels to give up control.

EXERCISES TO YIELD:

OBJECTIVE: TO FACILITATE FLEXIBILITY

That which is more malleable is superior to that which is hard metal. Control your life by going with the flow.

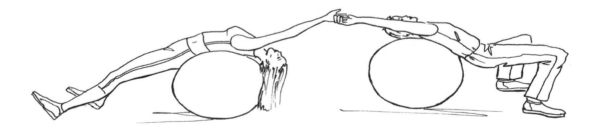

CORE STABILITY AND BALANCE
You will need a partner and 2 stability balls. Each of you lies back on a stability ball head to head, arms length apart and knees bent. Then reach out overhead and holding hands gently pull in an easy roll first towards one partner and then towards the other. As you pull in one direction your legs straighten, but the knees are supple and your back and head are supported on the ball, while your partner's legs are bent. Then roll back as your knees bend, while your partner stretches out on the ball. Aim for 10 rolls. You and your partner adapt to each other's pull.

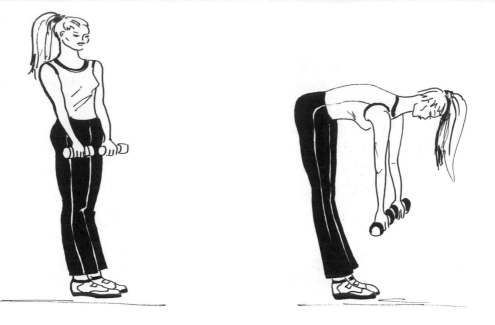

DEAD LIFTS

A straight leg dead lift holding (3,5,8,10 lb weights or a 12 lb bar) helps you to stretch your hamstrings, work your glutes and lower back as well as strengthen spinal alignment. If you grasp a bar or dumbbells, use an overhand grip and stand up straight. Then keeping your legs nearly locked, bend forward at the waist until your upper body is almost parallel with the floor. Hold your abdominals in tightly and make sure your back is flat. The weights or bar should be hanging arm's length below. Maintain tight abdominals, as you use the muscles in the back of your legs to return to the starting position. Tighten your glutes on the way up. Remember not to hunch your back. Do 3 sets of 8 repetitions gradually advancing to 15 repetitions per set along with heavier weights. As you lower, your upper body yields to your arms and as you rise, your back yields to your hamstrings.

YIELD WITH YOGA

To learn how to yield consider taking up *Hatha yoga* which provides a healthy regimen to build good body awareness along with flexibility. This keeps the spine healthy and every joint loose and free. Stretching poses can be done daily and are especially beneficial after weight training to promote longer and less bulky muscles. When "shopping" for a yoga class, find one that matches your needs: flexibility, balance, strength or meditation. It is a good idea to warm up for 5-10 minutes before class with light cardio on the stationary bike or by walking. Remember: never strain to get into a pose, or "force it." Stretching is never done to the point of pain, no matter what everyone else is doing in class. Pay attention to proper form and alignment. Practice deep abdominal breathing. Through deep stretching yoga postures cleanse the muscles of deposited stress hormones, improve circulation and gradually increase range of motion. *Stretch your body, stretch your mind.*

CHAPTER 18

TRAINING TO SHUT UP

Heard melodies are sweet, but those unheard are sweeter
John Keats

We grew up with the proverb, "Silence is golden." According to Zen philosophy when one attains true enlightenment, speech becomes unnecessary. Emily Dickinson wrote about the Godlike power of language, "A word said is never dead." One must be careful of spoken words; the implication is that it is safer not to speak. Silence is the polar opposite of speech, self-contained, listening as opposed to speaking, demonstrably doing. Talking is outgoing, action oriented, kinetic, and insistent. Silence rests contentedly with the inner self, at ease, attune to the universe, essentially a recipient of wisdom.

Ideally, life is a balance between these two states of being, the male-female components of our body, the yin and yang of our spiritual makeup. Often we cause trouble when we speak before we think, lash out in anger, declare our feelings to others who are not ready to hear them, brow beat them to submission and repeat our opinions as though constant assertion would make them true.

How often have we regretted hasty accusations, or comments blurted out, later to be followed with "I'm sorry." However, the words can never be unsaid, never forgotten. Our words cut like daggers, wound the heart and can kill another human being with an acerbic

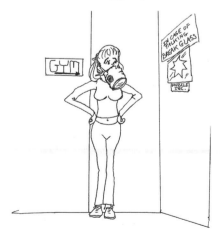

barb to his or her self-esteem. Sometimes in the heat of the moment our words offer false promises, phony compliments to ensure that we are well liked, or boast to impress others. We say things we don't mean which others take for truth. We need to think before we speak, keep silent until we have achieved equilibrium between our intellect and sensibility.

When we don't speak, we appear more intelligent and thoughtful. We mystify people who try to guess our thoughts, penetrate our being. Count your words and make them count! When we don't speak, we listen to others and learn to be genuinely interested in what they have to say. We leave our self-centered world to learn, absorbing their words to truly understand them. "Keep your cup empty, then it is useful," is a Zen proverb reminding even the most accomplished to be willing to listen and learn. One of my favorite Zen stories tells of a Western professor who visits a Japanese Master. His mission is to learn Eastern philosophy. However, when West meets East, the professor pontificates and describes his own accomplishments instead of listening. "Would you care to participate in a tea ceremony?" the Master asks. They sit down on mats and the Zen Master pours the tea and continues to pour the tea until it is overflowing in a stream on the floor. "Don't you see that my cup is overflowing?" shouts the professor. "Exactly, when the cup overflows, it does not hold the liquid," replies the Master. The professor learns that when you speak to show off, you do not listen, learn and retain. Another benefit to listening and pausing is that we make ourselves far less vulnerable to overreacting or speaking our minds too authoritatively when we are wrong.

Usually when we speak, it is to compel others to make them yield to our thinking. We need to learn to rest contentedly to just "be." When we give up control, we manifest it in our speech or non-speech, for we listen to other voices, other ideas. We need to be present and aware, noticing what is being said and often more importantly, what is *not* being said. Then we will paradoxically discover our inner voice, which is also silent and does not need to speak, yet needs to emerge.

On the training floor I have arrogantly boasted of my prowess with weight training or aerobic moves. "I don't have to stop now; I could do a hundred more!" "I really like this exercise. It's easy!" To which my trainer Frank with an "I'll teach you a lesson" look in the eye, would say, "Good, that's impressive: 100, 99, 98, 97..." or " That was only the warm-up, here do these squats now with eight pound weights exploding up into shoulder presses." I huff and puff, sweat raining down my forehead; Oh how I wish I hadn't opened my big mouth. "When will I learn to keep my mouth shut?" I ask sweetly and submissively, hoping Frank has lost count and forgiven my arrogance. "I don't know" is the answer uttered with a broad grin, "49, 48, come on, continue."

And when my muscles have ached because of words carelessly tripping off the tongue, since old patterns die hard, I vow to keep my mouth shut. There is no need to brag about our accomplishments. Actions speak louder than words!

MIND/BODY PRESCRIPTIONS:

Practice communicating silently. Listen with your eyes. Gaze into another person's eyes while you do not speak to him or her. Allow that person to speak freely. Study and learn. Do not ask any questions. What do you discover about that person? What do you discern about the meaning of the words? Are you able to focus on what that person is saying, or is your mind wandering to your own thoughts? Continue to be silent. Hold your gaze. Does the speaker continue to meet yours? Are you able to maintain your silence even if the speaker demands a response? Resist the temptation to reply verbally. Allow your silence to speak for you. Let the speaker infer your thoughts.

MEDITATION:

Sit with your palms facing up. Close your eyes and relax your body. Begin by visualizing your breath go in and go out. Then imagine an expansive meadow on a breezy spring day. You are drawn to a tall weeping willow that has small delicate leaves on yellow-green fronds. Notice how they dance in the wind. There are no human voices, only the wind in the willows. Listen carefully. The sounds you hear resemble words. Do not question. Do not request a repetition of the sounds. Instead simply listen. Continue to inhale and exhale. What emotions come up for you at this time? Listen in deep silence. Hear the wind in the willows again. Allow the sounds to penetrate your being. Can you make out the air borne words now? The wind affects everything around you. The long grasses sway. This natural music strikes a chord in your heart. Bring your complete attention to this time and place. You are present to your surroundings and your feelings: silent, secure and at ease. When you feel ready to return to your body, open your eyes and bring this quiet peaceful awareness to your life.

EXERCISES TO SHUT UP: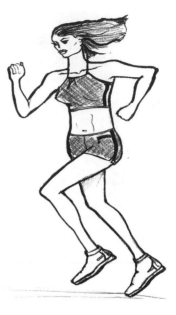

OBJECTIVE: ACTIVE STILLNESS TO CREATE FOCUS

SPRINTS

A sprint workout necessitates the runner to be fast and focused. One cannot run, breathe and talk at the same time. Stand on a basketball court, tennis court, boardwalk, or quiet road and explode out for about 120 feet; then walk back the same distance. When you sprint, be sure to lift your feet off the ground and cut through the air with your hands. Begin with 2 repetitions. Compete with yourself or a friend to increase speed. As you progress, do 4 to 8 repetitions and increase your distance by sprinting around the entire court and then walking it out.

STABILITY BALL

*Sit on a stability ball and center yourself to maintain balance. Lift your knee and still maintain your balance. Alternate legs. Keep your focus straight ahead to the horizon and hold abdominals in tightly. When you feel comfortable, you find yourself speaking as you lift and lower your legs. The next phase of the exercise is more complex. As you lift and lower your legs, hold a dumbbell in each hand (3, 5, or 8 lbs) and do biceps curls exploding up into a shoulder press. Please see chapter 3, **Training to Love Yourself** for a biceps curl. The biceps curl goes to a full hang and then contracts from the biceps muscle. The wrist rotates to face out and lifts up straight into a shoulder press (shown), rising from the elbows which are supple, not hyper-extended. One cannot speak as one strives to maintain balance, flow into the movements and lift the weights. As one leg goes up, a biceps curl and shoulder press are completed. Do a set of 8 repetitions on each side. As you advance, do 3 sets of 12, increasing the weight of the dumbbells.*

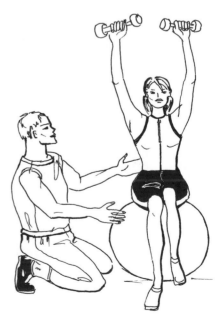

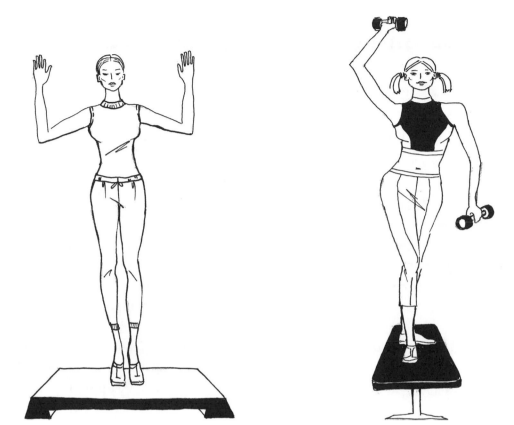

TARGETS LEGS, GLUTES AND SHOULDERS

*For a good cardio and strength training workout that keeps you silent, here are two variations. In the simpler version raise your hands as though you were being held up at gunpoint and step up and down a step or a bench. First do 8 repetitions starting on the right foot, then on the left. Do 3 sets. For a more advanced move, add stability pods to the step or use a bench and holding a weight in each hand (begin with 3 lb dumbbells advancing when this exercise gets easier to 5 lbs) laterally (sideways) step up and down the bench starting on the right foot. Then step up and down the bench facing front beginning with the left foot. Then do it on the right and finish by laterally stepping up and down the bench on the left foot. Do 8 repetitions per leg all around the bench—a total of 32. When that gets easier and you wish to add intensity, hold a weight down with your left hand as you laterally step up a bench with your left foot and raise your right arm concurrently into a shoulder press. Then facing forward step up 8 times on the right foot and then 8 times on the left foot as you do shoulder presses with **both** arms up. Conclude with lateral steps on the right foot and a left hand shoulder press. Again step up 8 times per leg all around the bench for a total of 32. Work your way up to 12 per leg for a total of 48. Aim for 3 sets.*

CHAPTER 19

TRAINING FOR DIVORCE

And when we close the curtains, oh,
We hold each other against that cold white sign
Of the way we all begin and end. Hello.
Good-bye is the only story
Martha Collins

In order to train for divorce, the mind and body must be connected to disconnect from the failing union. Because divorce uncouples the familiar, the safety net of our lives, even if it is a worn, frazzled, or constricting net, it is still what we know as opposed to the unknown. We fear change. Some of us feel that lightning has split our house in two. It crashes down while we watch it happen from a distance. We step carefully amidst the rubble of our relationship trying to find the remnant of the original foundation to rebuild the original self, no longer attached to a spouse. "Sometimes you take me over the top and sometimes you just push me right off!" We need to recover our self-esteem because we have seen ourselves reflected in our spouse's eyes and those eyes may have provided a distorted view. "He never made me feel like anything because he never felt like he was anything." We have to learn to break the habit, become independent and grow accustomed to being alone with ourselves.

PROBLEMS AND CHANGES

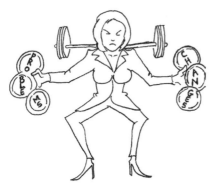

TAKE CONTROL

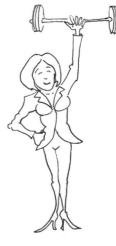

Many of us fear going unaccompanied to a movie or eating alone in a restaurant unless seated at the counter. We have to relearn to be quiet and still within, content with our own company and if not, work on ourselves, to raise self-esteem and accomplishment. Then we will realize that our original framework is still sound. At first one could get used to performing little activities alone, like going for a bike ride or a long walk. Once comfortable with this phase, one could go to the theatre, or visit a museum. The next step might be spending a weekend alone in a hotel room in the city or at a country inn. The mind is actively seeking to get reacquainted with new goals, or even forgotten goals of the single individual as opposed to the duo. During a marriage one partner's goal might have been unevenly shared by both, instead of blending the two separate individual goals, each discernable in his or her own right.

Unfortunately many divorces do not end in an amicable parting of the ways, resulting in angry words, hostility and vengeful threats and actions. When one partner lives in the dark about finances and does not have a job outside the home, the divorce process creates tension, fear and depression, as it highlights the weaker party. Therefore training the muscles as well as the mind provides a physical workout serving as an outlet for frustrations, providing the armor and self-esteem to enable a fledgling warrior to fight this uncivil civil war.

Uncoupling is a process. Therefore the workout must be a process, too; for example, martial arts is a good choice as the student progresses in stages. There can be no instant gratification. Painstakingly, movements are learned in a ritual dance flowing one into the other. Fighting utilizes both kinetic, rapid movements, and static contractions, for centered energy. One learns to see the self and an opponent as one, a complement. One absorbs the attack of the opponent and using his force, overcomes him.

An additional benefit that martial arts provides is that learning the *forms* of the dance is about learning to fight with awareness, grace and most importantly with self control. Forms teach the participant order and flow. When learning the forms, one attains a basic knowledge of punching and blocking. This combination of movements creates success in battle as opposed to a knockout punch. For in martial arts varied punches in rapid succession coupled with different types of kicks create speed, agility and surprise.

However, if rage is running high during divorce, martial arts might be too combative a workout for the amateur, escalating a battle instead of a settlement. The consummate martial artist does not seek violence. In fact he shuns it, for he arms himself in the art of fighting in order not to fight. He moves out of the way, or shows his power artfully, alerting the attacker to move away because he will be overpowered. He uses just enough force to subdue the enemy. If his life is threatened and these methods have not stopped the attack, then he will defend himself by unleashing full power. This self-control takes years of experience. Someone involved in highly charged divorce proceedings must exercise caution when beginning a martial arts program if he is prone to rage or violence. Physical aggression might make the participant mentally aggressive and uncompromising; otherwise, martial arts provides great training for confronting the "slings and arrows of outrageous fortune" in a peaceful manner!

Another process oriented ritual exercise is tai chi. It is a more passive and slow moving workout tapping into a person's "chi" or energy. The tai chi movements are definite as they create inner calm. When practicing the forms, the movements flow like a river and emanate from within. The principle is never to stop the chi's fluidity, the positive healthy energy. When one feels stressed, or enraged, his chi is dammed up unable to flow freely; either it will burst, exploding and destroying everything in its path, or through a series of slowly controlled exercises will become channeled, redirected to flow in a new, freer direction. The energetic rivers of life no longer impeded, move toward a newer, unblocked destination. This mind/body connection trains the divorced person to reconnect with life, as succinctly stated in the Chinese proverb: "Ten thousand rivers flow into the sea/ The sea is never full."

Another process-oriented exercise training both mind and body as well as promoting strength, flexibility and serenity, is yoga. Because of the tense divorce environment, its verbal and legal battles, yoga presents an option for moving meditation. Those who do not wish to perform the militant dance of martial arts, or the slow internal movements of tai chi, might prefer to perform active-stillness exercises that center one's power and energy. The various postures channel strength and endurance in both mind and body, yet teach flexibility. They prompt the participant to stretch beyond his limitations, thus stimulating self-improvement and accomplishment. Some yoga classes are held in a high heat environment of 105 degrees where the participant sweats out the toxins in his body as he strengthens his core muscles. Worthy to note: yoga widens the arteries and veins in the circulatory system, constricted by cholesterol deposits; therefore yoga is wonderful for those suffering from heart disease, or who wish to prevent it. Metaphorically and physically, yoga heals the heart.

The added benefit of martial arts, tai chi and yoga is that they are all non-competitive workouts that tap into the collective energy of the group. One progresses according to personal ability with improvement measured by personal accomplishment, not by the group's. Obviously when someone suffers through the divorce process, he or she is least likely to feel better in a competitive workout. However, in these exercises one emerges as an individual with group support in the backdrop. The sting of alienation that divorce triggers can be lessened in these classes because of the strong cerebral control and positive energy the group communicates in its movements and breathing techniques. A good follow-up would be a group meditation, offering a collective prayer for well being and balance. These classes help a newly uncoupled person find his or her inner strength, the individuality lost as part of a bad marital match, restoring the faith and courage to move forward.

The message in all three workouts is: *don't quit on yourself in class. If you do, you'll quit on something else pertaining to your life. Hold on to your will, for you will get over this painful period in your life. It is the attempt, the journey that matters. Small steps, giant gains.*

Specific muscles to be strength trained for divorce are the shoulders and back muscles. Uncoupling gives each member a cross to bear as God gives each one the strength to carry and endure the load. When back muscles are trained, posture is improved. We can stand taller and straighter, more proudly. A person who slouches, walks with stooped shoulders, is depressed, lacks self-esteem, or slouches throughout life, not doing his share of the workload.

Other important muscle groups to be trained for divorce are the quadriceps, hamstrings and calves strengthening our legs to help us move to the next place. If we don't move forward, we will be planted in the same place in our misery. We build up our leg muscles because they will carry us to our next happiness. Although a marriage of two minds and two bodies has failed, each member needs to explore and rediscover the delightful individual who previously existed by removing the shackles of the past. Each separated member needs to embrace the whole self before seeking another companion.

MIND/BODY PRESCRIPTIONS:

STEP ONE: TAKING CARE OF YOURSELF

Of course, you have to meditate regularly to find inner peace and perhaps, see a therapist or a support group for guidance, but the *superficial* is a good place to begin. When you start to care about yourself by eating right, working out and dressing the part, you project to the outside world a positive outlook. And the world always responds! Remember looking good is the best revenge.

STEP TWO: SUPPORT SYSTEM

Cultivate all your existing relationships, children and friends. If you become involved in another relationship, you might forget your friends. Remember lovers come and go, but true friends endure.

STEP THREE: SELF-DEVELOPMENT

If you don't have a job or never had one, get a job! Working and earning a paycheck gives you self-worth and independence. You never get a paycheck for being a housewife! Get trained in a new career and when you go out to work everyday to perform that new job, you will expand your world and meet new people.

MEDITATION:

In a quiet room sit with dignity, your palms face up resting on your thighs receptive to universal energy. Close your eyes and begin to breathe rhythmically. Inhale and exhale through your nose. Imagine that you are a complex, life-size jigsaw puzzle. There are hundreds of colorful pieces that fit together to create your image. See these pieces combining one by one. Notice how some fit together easily while others do not. Don't force any piece to fit. Continue to breathe and relax your heart. Allow the pieces to combine and recombine to form a complete picture. They touch and pull apart until they fit together easily. When all the pieces are connected, observe the puzzle. What is the dominant color? What picture do you see? And how does that picture make you feel? Be with that emotion for a moment. Slowly leave the backdrop to emerge seamlessly as a three-dimensional being. You have put yourself together. Although you are composed of many complex pieces, you are one and feel at peace with this oneness. Return to your body and slowly open your eyes. Smile as the new you awakens.

EXERCISES FOR DIVORCE:

OBJECTIVE: TAKING CONTROL TO MOVE FORWARD

SQUATS WITH A BROOM SYMBOLIZE THE BURDEN WE CARRY AS A RESULT OF OUR DIVORCE

SQUATS
Stand with feet shoulder width apart, knees slightly bent. Place a broom or a weighted bar (for a more advanced move) lightly on your shoulders behind your neck. Bend your knees as though sitting back with your glutes on an imaginary chair. Remember to keep your chin up. **Important:** *Keep your heels flat on the floor as you move your glutes to the rear. Do* **not hyperextend** *knees over toes. Return to the starting position. Do 10-15 repetitions per set, building up to 3 sets. When that gets too easy, do three sets of 25.*

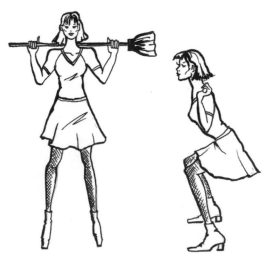

POWERFULLY RESTRAINED, ACTIVELY STILL, TO CONNECT
TO THE WARRIOR WITHIN

WARRIOR I

Begin from a standing position. Step 3 feet to the side with the right foot pointing so that it is perpendicular to the left. Bend the right knee while keeping the left foot strong and straight. Your pelvis faces toward your right foot. Your arms are raised overhead beside your ears, palms together. Open your heart center (your chest). For a more advanced position, drop your hips 3 inches lower. Hold for 5 deep breaths, inhaling and exhaling through the nose. Notice: when you inhale there is an expansion of the body and when you exhale, allow all the air out of your abdomen which contracts from the navel to the back. If you feel any resistance upon exhaling, say quietly to the self, "let go." Do 3 repetitions. Switch legs and repeat.

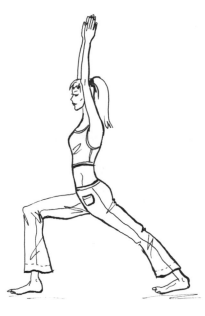

WARRIOR II

Begin with the same stance as Warrior I, but make it one foot wider. Now square off your hips by turning your pelvis ever so slightly to the left. Arms extend out straight shoulder height. Gaze over the right shoulder and hold this position for 5 deep breaths. Look ahead to your future (symbolized by your right shoulder) as you look away from the past (symbolized by your left shoulder), yet keep the lessons learned. Do 3 repetitions. Then switch legs and repeat.

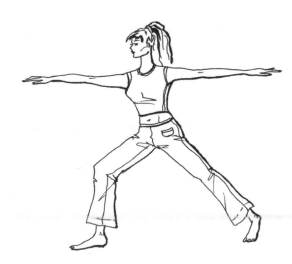

BOBBING AND WEAVING TO DUCK THE BLOWS OF RECRIMINATION

BOB AND WEAVE

Squat in a horse stance, 3 feet apart, knees bent, heels firmly planted on the ground. Keep your hands, palms facing out, next to your ears to be used as a marker since there is no real bar to duck under. Shift your body weight from the right heel to the left heel ducking below an imaginary bar as though you were lifting to the other side. Use your legs. Push off your heels to propel you up and down. This move tightens quads and glutes. Do one set of 25 repetitions working up to 3 sets of 50 repetitions.

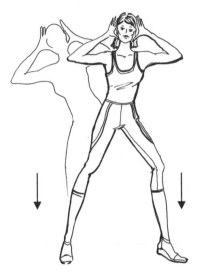

ADD A MEDICINE BALL

For a more advanced move hold a weighted medicine ball (up to 12 lbs) in front of your chest as you bob and weave under an imaginary bar. This move is more aerobic to help you burn fat as well as to add weight to your muscles for sculpting. Begin with a set of 25 repetitions and work your way up to 3 sets of 50 repetitions.

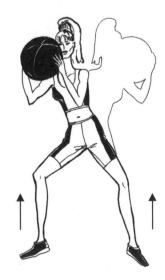

LUNGES STRENGTHEN QUADS, GLUTES AND HAM STRINGS TO HELP US WALK TO OUR NEXT HAPPINESS

LUNGES

Stand with feet together shoulders back and head up. Step forward with the right foot bending both knees. Force your body weight through the heel. The right knee is at a 90 degree angle making sure that the front knee does not extend over the toe. The left knee is bent to the floor, almost touching. Keeping the front foot flat on the floor, step back with the right foot to the start position. Repeat with the left foot, alternating legs to a set of 10 repetitions per leg. Work your way up to 3 sets of 25 per leg. For greater intensity, hold two 5-8 lb dumbbells. For a more advanced movement do walking lunges. Beginning with the right leg, step forward coming into a lunge; then walk forward with the left foot and step into a lunge. Your goal is to walk back and forth across a room. For the most advanced move, if your divorce is especially difficult, do walking lunges with two 5-8 lb dumbbells. Remember with focused determination you will once again move forward.

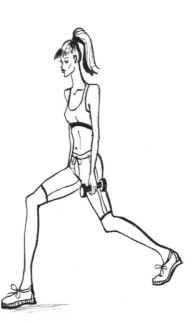

TAI CHI, QI-GONG OR MARTIAL ARTS: A PROCESS ORIENTED WORKOUT

"Knocked down to the Ground
Rise Gracefully
Stand Firm
Open Heart"

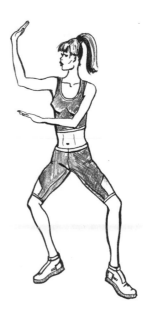

CHAPTER 20

TRAINING FOR DISAPPOINTMENT

There is no disappointment we endure
One half so great as that we are to ourselves
Philip James Bailey

Everyone has a different threshold for disappointment just as we all have a different threshold for pain. Some of us are always waiting "for the other shoe to drop," while others are surprised, even amazed, that things did not go their way. Some of us prepare for disappointment, so as not to be *too disappointed* when "it" happens. While others cheerily expect everything to work out and if it doesn't, they experience an emotional drop, but for the most part they feel happy. We have all experienced disappointment at work or in relationships when the goals we set for ourselves were not achieved, or our significant others did not fulfill our lofty expectations.

JUMP FROM YOUR LAST DISAPPOINTMENT TO LAND ON YOUR NEXT SUCCESS

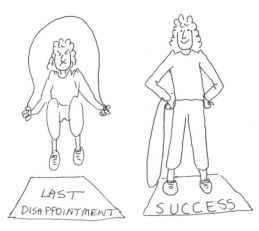

Disappointment is accompanied by feelings of rejection and failure. However, it is important to experience disappointment, even though it means that we have failed. Failure can be beneficial because we grow and learn to do better. Some of the best successes in life are derived from failed dreams. We do not have to fall down; Dr. Bernie Siegel reminds us that we can "fall up." When we feel dejected because we have failed, disappointed in ourselves, we need to regain composure, return to the self. When we fail, the universe is sending us a message, a signal that we need to analyze and redirect our energies for new developments and new successes. As Dolly Parton puts it, *"There can be no rainbow without some rain."*

Setbacks in life compel us to look inward at our limitations, as a preparation to take a leap of faith in ourselves to develop our capabilities. Sometimes we become impatient, frustrated that we cannot succeed as quickly or as overtly as we would wish. However, by working slowly, methodically, we can move on to our next success. Our disappointments serve as a contrast to intensify the sweetness of accomplishment.

Suspicion and self-doubt impede our forward movement to success. Often we carry these two emotions as baggage along with our disappointment. When we do not trust ourselves to do better, or others to help us do better, or the universe to guide us in doing better, we block our energy flow and become stagnant. When we suspect our friends and our lovers, it is because we fear they will disappoint us. Our suspicions prepare us for the worst. Why do we anticipate disappointment? We do not feel worthy of love or greatness. We project unto others what is lacking in ourselves. In essence we are bracing ourselves for dramas that may never take place except in our suspicious imaginations. All this stems from a fundamental lack of self-esteem. We are implying that our friends and lovers could not possibly find us attractive, substantial and delightful for very long. For once they spend enough time with us, the magic will undoubtedly wear off. Ultimately, these suspicions which kiss our lovers' lips or whisper into the ears of employers will create a self-fulfilling prophecy, alienating and prodding others to disappoint us because of the negative energy we emit. My friend, a former martial artist, serves as an example. Recently, he showed me his misshapen knuckle, a reminder of damaging self-doubt. During a competition he had to punch through a number of wooden boards, which he had performed successfully many times. However, this time he experienced a fleeting moment of self-doubt and thus broke his knuckle instead of the boards.

When we fail in our relationships or our endeavors, we need to transform ourselves to be able to succeed. We need to experience our failure, learn from it, and perhaps hardest of all, not to judge or condemn it. Do we judge a rock or fallen tree trunk in the road? When we realize that an obstacle sits on a necessary path in the journey of life, we can be determined and optimistic about finding a solution. Sometimes to get in touch with our inner radar, our intuition, we need to fail and suffer in order to purify ourselves, strip away the clutter to rediscover what is primal and vital. However, that does not mean that we should suppress the pain of disappointment. By feeling the pain, we mourn the loss in order to release the old pattern of behavior or negative thinking. Yield to the disappointment to overcome it; don't struggle against it. Once we change the picture in our head, affirmatively, we will change our energy. Our worst enemies are our own negative thoughts. We must try to have compassion and love for the self.

Ultimately, the key to shedding disappointment is simple to render, but complex to attain: to lower our expectations. Frequently, we set up unrealistic expectations for the self and others, causing internal stress and an impediment to contentment. Instead of focusing on and desiring what we don't have, *we must strive to want what we do have.*

MIND/BODY PRESCRIPTIONS:

◆ Recite or write down an affirmation for a specific endeavor. Say *it*; believe *it* and *it* will happen.

◆ When you feel the cold hands of failure, think warm thoughts to warm your muscles, your heart and soul. The warmth will create calmness and a soothing state of mind, like a cup of hot chocolate in front of the fireplace.

◆ Believe that you are headed on the path that you are meant to be on. Every obstacle you encounter is meant for you to overcome.

◆ Improve your strong points to outweigh your limitations.

◆ Learn to live in the present. Accept yourself for what you are now, not what you once were.

MEDITATION:

Sit with dignity palms facing up. Close your eyes and look up towards your eyebrows. Inhale and exhale. Relax your breaths. Find yourself standing alone in a vast room. Outside, darkness is fast approaching. The room has a tall ceiling, a polished wooden floor, tall windows and no furniture. The walls are bare. You notice there is no fixture to illuminate the room. How will you be able to see? There are no distractions here and you are alone with yourself. Take a moment to reflect. Your body will help bring awareness to your mind. Notice any sensations in your body. Does your neck suddenly feel stiff? Does your stomach feel tight now? If so, note that your body is sending you a message. Experience this message. What does it symbolize for you? Night has fallen and you realize that you have no remaining, natural light. A feeling of disappointment washes over you. See what comes up for you now. Relax your breaths. Perhaps you feel that there is someone you are disappointing. It might be you or someone close to you-- perhaps both. Now imagine another possibility. There in the far corner of the room stands an antique oil lamp on a pedestal table. Next to the lamp, rest long tapered matches and an oil can. Watch yourself fill the lamp with oil. Light it. You feel restored with new positive sensations. Now that you can see again, allow the light to absorb your disappointment. When you are ready, open your eyes. Remember: like the lit oil lamp, your dreams are difficult to extinguish.

EXERCISES FOR DISAPPOINTMENT:

OBJECTIVE: TO FAIL AND THEN SUCCEED

Try new things that will test you for the first time. You will struggle and then learn to be proficient through practice. Jumping rope is one of the most frustrating exercises to learn. Jumping rope well takes a lot of patient practice to achieve good coordination. It is a wonderful cardio workout, burns a great deal of calories, is effective in preventing osteoporosis because of its gravity-oriented movement and strengthens the hamstrings and quadriceps in the process. Begin in short bursts of seconds building up to minutes. Because the equipment is light-weight, you can carry a jump rope with you to work or on vacation. An added spiritual benefit is that it will train you to leap over your setbacks, inspiring you with a leap of faith in yourself. *Jump over your next hurdle to land on your feet.*

Another exercise for facing your next challenge is taking your first step class or dance class in Salsa or Hip Hop. You feel that everyone else knows the visual cues and the calls, except you. Disappointed that you look clumsy, your timing is off and you can't remember the choreography. Keep taking the same class for a month. You not only succeed, but feel at ease and unafraid to learn new steps. You stand near the instructor in front of the room instead of all the way in the back.

When I weight train and have collapsed at the last push-up, or fallen on my butt doing triceps dips off a bench, Frank, my trainer, barks, "We don't end with failure, reach in there and give me one more! We end with our last success." And guess what? I am able to do one more. That's a good less in life!

THE MEDITATION WALK
- ◆ I CAN
- ◆ I WILL
- ◆ I DO
- ◆ !!

THE MEDITATION WALK

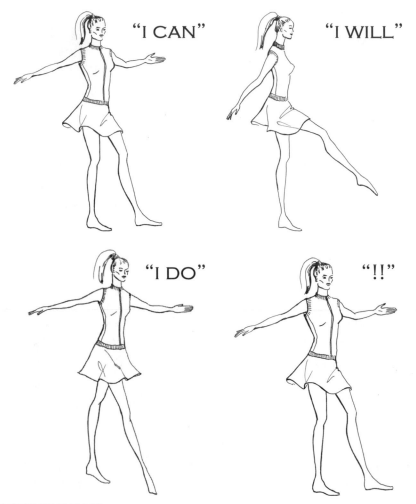

"I CAN"

"I WILL"

"I DO"

"!!"

QI-GONG WALK

*This Meditation Walk is adapted from Qi-Gong—gentle internal and external movements to realign (chi) energy and well- being. Begin this walk with your chest open and your arms slightly extended out behind you. Point your toe forward as though you were a ballerina. Take a step forward. Then do three more steps moving gracefully forward. Next imagine that as you take a first step, there is a number one directly under foot. Step on it. Then walking in the same fashion as before, step on number two, three and four. Now, imagine on your first step forward that you are stepping on a word, "I can." Then on your second step, "I will." Your third step, "I do." Your last step, "!" Step purposefully on each word and say each word aloud at the same time: **I can, I will, I do, !!** I can means potential. **I will** means affirmation. **I do** means implementation. !! means with eagerness. The speed with which you walk suggests the stage you have reached. In other words, the faster pace implies that you are on the level of implementation, rather than potential. If you take it to a jog, you have transcended your disappointment.*

CHAPTER 21

TRAINING TO HANDLE MONEY

Money, which represents the prose of life,
And which is hardly spoken of in parlors
Without an apology, is in its effects and laws,
As beautiful as roses
Ralph Waldo Emerson

Money can be a great liberator, freeing us to do the things we really want to do with our lives, or money can imprison us if we sell our souls to make it for status. Is it a means or an end? Money introduces ambiguity into our lives. We might feel guilty if we possess it, or unsuccessful, unhappy if we don't.

In a superficial world, a material world, money is used as a measuring stick. Purchase-power, designer clothes, fancy cars and affluent homes make us feel accomplished or do they? Some of us feel pressured to make more money to preserve this flamboyant lifestyle because we are competitive with the friend or neighbor who will always have a fancier home or car. We begin to worry if the stock market goes down; after all, we could lose money when we invest, or lose the ability too keep making it. No one has unraveled the mystery of the Midas touch, or the length of time one possesses it.

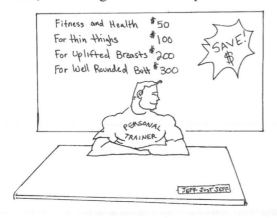

When money runs your life, you have to wonder: am I happier accumulating money? Do I sacrifice my creative expression for money? Am I in a job that makes money, but I don't like what I do? Am I driven to make money to compel my significant other to stay with me? When money runs your life and you are not true to your core, or when you spend too much of your life working for it, rather than having it work for you, happiness becomes elusive.

What would happen if you found a job you enjoy without worrying about having "enough" money? Perhaps, your creative energy would flow and it would act like a magnet to bring money to you. When you are excited and enthusiastic about what you do, you will ultimately attract money. This may sound far-fetched, but there is some inexplicable connection in the universe between positive energy and making money.

When you flow with abundant positive energy, you make money. When you are stingy, uncharitable with yourself as well as with others, you lose money. Money becomes an extension of your spiritual identity, a reflection of the self you have become. People are valued for their actions just as a business is valued by its profits. How you handle money reveals your personality. You need to reflect if you are stingy with your feelings, or if you generously give of yourself and of your time. You can sell out those on the lower rungs of the social ladder or your friends for selfish desire, or you can *invest in friendships*.

Often you hear derisive remarks about *new* money. Middle class or poor folk who have made a considerable amount of money are mocked, referred to as hillbillies because of their lack of financial etiquette. Old money is associated with subtlety and polish while new money drips with jewelry and a more ostentatious lifestyle. Nevertheless both breeds are pointed to with the same assessment: "You know how many millions he has?" The differences in demeanor and speech are merely a superficial veneer. The bottom line is people evaluate how much money one has and how he can be cajoled into spreading the wealth. It doesn't matter what one does to make money, only that he possesses it.

Is that how we want to be remembered or described? Is that our contribution to this earth? When money defines us, it obscures our self-expression, our inner self.

Not having money drives us to work hard because we feel pressured, self-induced or social, to prove our self-worth. We feel anxious, moody, exhausted as we struggle to prove our inner value. Sometimes the process becomes counterproductive. The harder we work, the less money we have as prices inflate and homes and cars loom above our reach. How humorous and simplistic to label people: middle class, lower class or upper class, based on an accumulation of possessions! Just as money should not define a person who has it, money should not define a person who does not have it.

I would rather see people labeled as teachers and students. We are always one or the other with different people: students with much to learn about life and teachers with much to share about our life experiences.

In training to handle money we need to respect the Puritan ethic about reaping what we sow. However, we need to understand that the harvest we reap is not the money itself, but the improvement it can bring to our spirit: the joy of living. Greed, stinginess and betrayal diminish our self-expression. The tree is recognized by its fruit and the fruits we bear emerge from the flowering of our personalities, validating ourselves by fulfilling good dreams and longings. Money is a facilitator.

If we look to the moral teachings of mythology, we learn never to sell out our inner selves for money. The Midas touch turned the king's most beloved daughter into a golden statue. To value money above our spiritual well being or our relationships with others is to lose our self-worth in the process. Ultimately, we are all going in the same direction on the graph of life. Kings and paupers face the same fate, for death is a great equalizer. Our immortality lies in our ability to love our fellow man releasing positive energy and harmony into the universe. This energy is stored in the hearts of the people whose lives we touch.

Money is not the root of all evil. We are the root of all evil when we do not honor ourselves or others for spiritual values.

MIND/BODY PRESCRIPTIONS:

SELF-WORTH

If you have defined your self worth based on your bank account, here are some exercises to follow.

- Balance your own checkbook. This will help you organize and create balance in your life.
- Make a security investment on your own. Feeling secure does not come from another. You must "invest" in what makes you feel secure.
- Take a loan from a bank rather than borrow from a friend or family. Establish your independent being.
- Go for a walk in the country. Observe animals in their natural habitat and how they live without money.
- Do volunteer work with cancer patients. Ask them about their views on money.
- Read books on Zen philosophy and Metaphysics to simplify and intensify your existence.
- Plant a garden. See how hard work earns you a profit.

MEDITATION:

Sit with dignity, your palms facing up. Close your eyes and begin breathing rhythmically. Relax your breaths. Imagine yourself on a lush island in the Pacific. Inhale the warm breeze and fragrant flowers. Exhale your material value system. You walk barefoot in the powdery sand along indigo waters to find local inhabitants. Many smiling faces greet you. However, you do not speak their language, nor do they speak yours. How do you feel? You observe that they are dressed simply and naturally. You look down at your own formal clothes. Experience the feelings that come up for you. The natives invite you into a hut. It is simple and bare. You are asked to sit in a circle and drink a ritual tea. The brew is hot and made of a natural herb. You drink it along with the others. Feel the warm herb permeate your body.

Everyone holds hands in a circle of friends. Experience the love and the happiness for a few moments. You observe that material possessions are virtually nonexistent on this island, but love abounds all around. Happiness is palpable in the air. Touch it and hold its energy between your hands for a moment. When you are ready, return to reality. Gradually, open your eyes bringing warmth and love into your daily existence. Let this natural feeling remain with you and guide you in all endeavors.

EXERCISES TO HANDLE MONEY:

OBJECTIVE: TO REALIZE YOUR INNER WORTH

- ♦ *If you pay more money to your personal trainer, will that buy you bigger muscles and greater endurance? Look around your aerobics class and see if the wealthiest is the most graceful.*
- ♦ *If you experience stress in the form of lower back pain, often it is a direct result of anxiety about a money matter.*

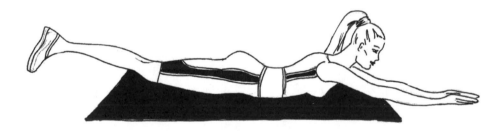

SUPERMAN

*For a lower back exercise, do the superman. Lie down on your abdomen with arms alongside you. Begin lifting your legs off the floor a few inches and hold for 5-10 seconds and lower. Then lift your shoulders off the floor and extend your arms out in front of you lifting them a few inches off the floor and hold for 5-10 seconds. For the most **advanced** version lift your legs and extend your arms out in front of you simultaneously and hold this position for 5- 10 seconds. Aim for 3 repetitions.*

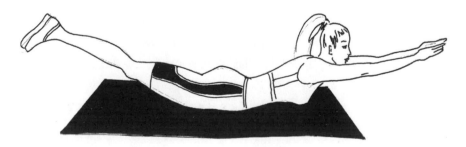

THE ABDOMINAL WHEEL

To strengthen your core, your shoulders and your lower back, try the abdominal wheel. Because I am an avid gardener, the motion of the abdominal wheel reminds me of plowing a field or making a furrow. Gardeners know how to reap the fruits of their labor. Go down on your knees as you hold the wheel, overhand grip on both sides. Holding your abs in tightly, roll out straight and extend fully as far as you can go. The wheel guides you. Your abdominals do not touch the floor at the fullest extension. Roll back. Try to do 5-8 repetitions initially. As you progress, aim for 3 sets of 8-10 repetitions.

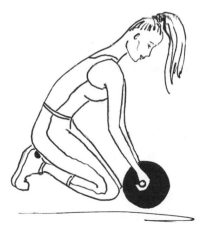

ABDOMINALS WITH A MEDICINE BALL

Do sit-ups while holding a weighted medicine ball over your chest. Feel as though you hold the world in your hands. When you crunch up, come off the shoulders, press your back into the floor, hold your abdominals in tightly, exhale. Return to the floor, but do not touch it with your shoulders. Aim for 10 repetitions. As you progress, increase the weight of the medicine ball and do 25 repetitions.

EXERCISES
MONEY CAN'T BUY

Inevitably, we are confronted by life situations that require us to be heroic both internally and physically. Money cannot bail us out. Status becomes meaningless. We need to recruit our muscles and third eye concentration. We need to believe in ourselves. For both men and women physical training has created muscles that save lives. To many the following responses to emergencies may seem Herculean, or supernatural. We have seen on TV how a man lifts a car off a trapped friend due to an adrenalin rush. However, if you have been strength training consistently, there is no magic here, only the will and the strong muscles to act out the mind's bidding. Visualize the action; then do it.

♦ *Squatting with a weighted barbell has strengthened quadriceps, hamstrings and glutes. If we needed to, we could carry a friend to safety slung over our shoulders, knees bent.*

♦ *Having trained at the cable row machine, back and biceps have been strengthened. We could pull a drowning person to shore.*

♦ *Having lifted at the bench press, chest, shoulders and triceps have been strengthened to lift fallen debris off our chest while we are pinned there under it.*

♦ *Doing chin-ups to strengthen back and biceps will enable us to pull ourselves up as we dangle from a precipice.*

♦ *Doing wide grip dips which strengthen chest and triceps will enable us to free ourselves from a car wreckage as we lift out before a possible explosion.*

♦ *The way we respond to an emergency reveals who we are, our true breeding and inner worth.*

CHAPTER 22

TRAINING FOR ROMANCE

Men always want to be a woman's first love...
We women have a more subtle instinct about things.
What we like is to be a man's last romance
Oscar Wilde

Because our sexuality is an expression of the life force, we are sensual creatures from childhood to old age. Sex is conceived in the brain and the mind is the most erotic organ in our bodies. There we fantasize about lovers, encounters and potential lovers and encounters, as well as unattainable lovers and encounters. Our minds interpret the sensual stimuli the body brings. Together mind and body merge with another mind and body for mutual satisfaction, mystical union, the life force and serene pleasure. Mystics believe that lovemaking creates a larger over-soul consisting of a mixture of the two separate individual souls that hover in ecstasy outside both lovers' bodies. *The Songs of Solomon* develop the allegory of the sensual love between a man and a woman as an expression of God's embracing love for mankind and our longing for that spiritual embrace. We are in love with another because we really want to connect to Divine love.

However, our innate sensuality can be modified, or suppressed by upbringing, religion, experiences with significant others, jobs and self-esteem. Our first love affair begins with the self, which is translated into auto-erotic experiences in childhood. Children are narcissists, self-involved in their pleasures and comforts and when they don't get their needs met, they know how to cry out for them. Children are uninhibited and don't experience shame until we teach them, reminiscent of Adam and Eve who grew ashamed of their nakedness. Sometimes we do such a good job teaching our children modesty and proper behavior that they grow up to be sexually inhibited, repressing their desires as dirty, not communicating personal needs to partners as they sacrifice their inner selves to be "good."

"NO, DON'T TURN ON THE LIGHT!"

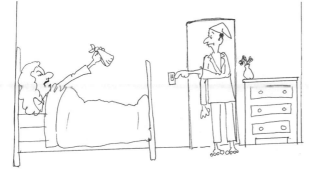

Therefore the first step towards getting reacquainted with our innate sexuality, our un-inhibited selves, is to look at ourselves naked in the mirror. Few of us would say, "Great body! How lucky for my mate! What a privilege to lie in bed next to me!" That's the source of our problem right there. If one doesn't like the self, or consider her body beautiful, then the negativity inevitably transmits itself to her lover and in bedroom performance. "I want to do it with the light on, honey." A gasp is heard, "Oh, no. Don't turn on the light!" "But I want to see you. I want to look at you. I wish there were a mirror on the ceiling." A cough is heard. "What's the matter, honey?" "I feel like I'm choking." However, men don't scrutinize their bodies the way women do. "I think I look damn good," he smiles at his image in the mirror as he sucks in his gut and makes a muscle with his arm.

If you don't like the way you look, no one else will either because true beauty emanates from the inside out. Your joy is diminished because you have lost your self-esteem in the bedroom. Far too busy covering up, ashamed of the body parts you are not satisfied with, you are not immersed in the moments of pleasure. How can you be open to the experience when you feel sexually unattractive?

The solution is obvious. The first step is to dress for success. Lingerie and heels go a long way to create mystery, sensuality and besides they cover up a lot of dietary indiscretions. Wearing a costume creates wit and excitement: cow girl, handyman, French maid, belly dancer, doctor, policeman etc. Camouflage works in military strategies and in the battle of the sexes the object is to take live prisoners.

Step two is to find a position that shows off your body in a more flattering angle. Lying prone on your back causes your abdominals to flatten. If you feel that your thighs are flabby, lifting your legs in the air tightens them and elongates the leg. If you like your butt best of all, then do an about face.

Step three takes the longest, but is the most lasting solution. Improve the body parts that displease you. Hard work and commitment will be reflected in the mirror. Working with a personal trainer to provide an intelligent program incorporating strength training and an aerobic workout will ensure steady improvement and a balanced fitness program. Classes in aerobics as well as in body sculpting also provide guidance and motivation along with group energy. Eating right and drinking plenty of water based on individual metabolism speeds up the process and improves skin tone.

Working out regularly helps you feel better about yourself as energy levels and endorphins rise as your appearance improves. And when you feel attractive and confident, others are magnetically drawn to you. Your happiness is irresistible, fueling others.

Also, strength training creates more testosterone in the body for both males and females. Testosterone increases libido in both sexes. Another benefit of weight lifting is increased blood flow to the sexual organs. The body is primed to perform like a well-tuned instrument. All that is necessary is a significant other to help the brain interpret the sensory signals through romance. That is where a romantic evening consisting of dinner with scented candles, wine, and music culminates in a bedroom dance.

Once you grow pleased with your appearance, the invention in your lovemaking will increase, as will the joy you bring to it. The light that shines on your bed will no longer intimidate you, but will now emanate from within to create intimacy and fulfillment.

MIND/BODY PRESCRIPTIONS:

BE INVENTIVE

- Present your lover with love coupons for redeemable kisses.
- Leave a trail of your clothes from the front door to the bedroom culminating with a love poem on his or her pillow.
- Play some romantic golden oldies from the decade of your youth.
- In the middle of a party whisper to your lover, "you're the most beautiful person here."
- Gaze into your lover's eyes with a penetrating look, especially when doing mundane chores together.
- Give your lover a hug from the opposite direction that you normally hug.

MEDITATION:

Sit comfortably with palms facing up. Close your eyes and breathe. Inhale and exhale to your own rhythm. See yourself exploring a verdant green countryside filled with delicately scented wildflowers. Let yourself experience this landscape using all your senses. As you continue down the path, you notice a card lying face down. Curiously, you bend down to pick it up. Your name is on the card and so you open it. Inside is a love poem. After reading it several times, although the card is unsigned, you know who wrote the poem. You continue down the path feeling as though someone is guiding you. Listen to the sounds of a horse drawn carriage. Suddenly it stops in front of you. The door opens and you enter to sit on tufted red velvet without asking any questions about the destination. Safe and secure, loved and special, you trust this journey. As hard as it is to open your eyes, return to your space. Bring these romantic feelings into your daily life. If you are receptive to romance, it will happen.

EXERCISES FOR ROMANCE: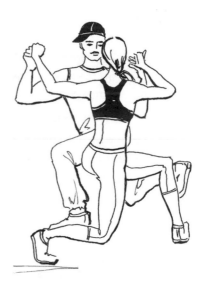

OBJECTIVE: TO FEEL ATTRACTIVE

Exercise together to make sure that your blood is pumping and that your libido is in sync. Go home and shower together, sensually. Dry off with hot towels that just came out of the dryer.

CROSS LUNGES

Do cross lunges together as you hold hands timing your exercise like a dance. Make sure to push off from the heel of your leading bent knee while your other leg bent at the knee in a 90 degree angle almost touches the floor. Your pelvis turns to face your partner. Your glutes, quads and hamstrings are tight. To move across the floor use the leg behind you to cross as your front leg lunges to the opposite side of your partner. Do 8 repetitions moving in one direction. Reverse your legs and direction; repeat for 8 repetitions. Aim for as many as your partner can persuade you to do. At the conclusion for added intensity, remain standing, drop hands and bring your legs in the cross lunge position closer to stand in curtsy position facing one another (not shown). *Go up and down rooting your front heel into the ground as the leg behind you helps you maintain balance. Do 8 repetitions. Switch legs and repeat. This is a polite and powerful way to end the dance.*

TANDEM LUNGES

*For another romantic variation of the traditional lunge, hold your partner's hand, right hand-left hand and do 8 stationary lunges coming forward on opposite knees. Remember to tighten your glutes and to lower your back leg **almost** to the ground. Do not let your knee hyperextend over your toes. Switch sides and do 8 repetitions. Aim for 3 complete sets of 10-12 repetitions. A rose between the teeth adds weight and increases romantic intensity.*

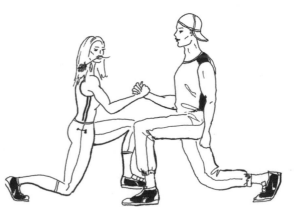

PARTNER GUIDED SQUATS

Squats take on a more sensual meaning as your partner guides you up and down in squat position your glutes lowering into an imaginary bucket. Push off your heels. Keep your back straight and do not hunch forward. Because your partner holds your hand, you can go lower and the lower you go, the more you target your glutes. You feel secure that he won't drop you and so you develop trust for each other. Your partner determines intensity and tempo by the pressure of his touch. Aim for 3 sets of 12-15. If you widen your stand with your toes pointing out, you will target your inner thighs. Aim for 3 sets of 12-15.

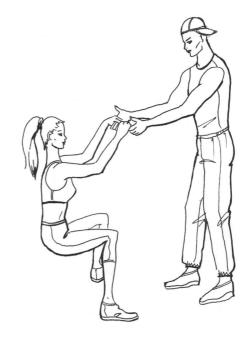

TARGETS OBLIQUES

Stand back to back as you pass a weighted medicine ball to each other in a continuous circular motion. You become one as you synchronize your body movements to work in harmony. Pass and receive the ball with one hand up on top and the other under the ball. Aim for 25 repetitions. As this gets easier, use a heavier ball (up to 14 lbs) and aim for 3 sets of 25 repetitions. This exercise works your obliques to give you a tapered waist that enhances your form.

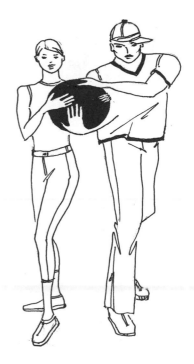

CHAPTER 23

TRAINING TO BE VULNERABLE

To be or not to be
Shakespeare, Hamlet

The word, vulnerable, connotes weakness, open to attack. The subject of vulnerability inevitably arises in any discussion about love relationships. Once you and your partner have been romantic several times, then what? The next step is soul searching. Will he or she respect my thinking, weaknesses and all? Since many of us strive to feel empowered, vulnerability appears to contradict this desirable state. However, ironically in order to feel in control, one has to know what vulnerability feels like. Empowerment does not imply controlling another person. Empowerment stems from the self and shows contentment with the self, not domination of another. When we develop self-esteem, appreciate our worth, we are not insecure about voicing our feelings. We have demonstrated that we are powerful enough to reveal ourselves. When we open up, though, we want and expect acceptance, not judgment. After all, if we have revealed our true feelings, shouldn't we be rewarded? However, sometimes we get the unexpected, *criticism*, or a negative answer. Therefore being vulnerable means taking a risk, facing the possibility of rejection. If we do not love ourselves enough to honor our authentic feelings, then we cannot be vulnerable to another person. Instead we hide, or pretend. Of course, we can never be rejected if we suppress our emotions or build a wall around ourselves. But then what are we *not* experiencing?

DON'T JUDGE YOUR FEELINGS

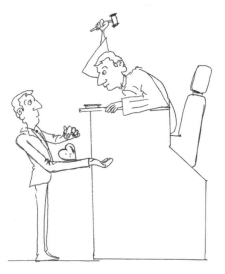

We will never know true happiness unless we let our inner light emanate. We will never experience the highs and the lows of life. The same applies to projects at work, or artistic endeavors. If we do not display them, they can never be rejected, but then they can never be appreciated either. We condemn ourselves to live in ambiguity and doubt: What if, could have...

One example of vulnerability that makes even a person with reasonably good self-esteem feel the beads of cold sweat and a dry mouth is public speaking. The speaker at the podium trembles at the thought that the audience might criticize his ideas along with his delivery. "If I tell a joke to warm up my audience, what if no one laughs?" "What if people yawn or talk among themselves during my presentation?" It takes hard work to overcome the fear of public speaking. First one must explore why he feels insecure about his perceptions: Are they revolutionary and controversial? Are they well researched? Is everyone in the room a genius? By objectively evaluating one's skills, the speaker can work through the obstacles. The vulnerable state of self-exploration can be truly liberating! Any flaws in reasoning and presentation can be fixed. A speech can be rewritten and delivery can be practiced with friends. At the podium the speaker hears a thundering applause and is invited to speak again.

Similarly, it is all right to admit at a job interview that we have no prior experience. Remember we can express our readiness to learn and eagerness to work hard to compensate. However, if we are afraid of being vulnerable at a job interview and don't even go, then we will not get the job anyway. In the worst case scenario, if we are rejected, new strength and resolve can be achieved because of the interview process, guiding us to better performance at other interviews, new opportunities. We can take consolation in gaining experience at interviewing. Eventually everybody gets that first job.

Vulnerability can lead to happiness in love because it is paradoxically a first step towards strengthening the ego. For example, a lover mirrors the internal self. If we are underdeveloped in a personality trait, we tend to find a significant other with the same problem. If we are not exploring ourselves, completing ourselves, but rather looking for another to do so, "you make me so happy," we are parasites in our love relationships, or addicts letting neediness run our lives. We have a crack in the foundation of our own ego system. When we have made ourselves vulnerable to ourselves, by digging deep inside to learn about our layers, our fears, only then are we ready to connect with another. We have to pay attention to ourselves before we can pay attention to a lover. If our spirit aches, let us look to a lover to help heal us, not to complete us. And a lover heals us through his support of our personal excavation.

Once we understand ourselves better, respect who we are, making ourselves vulnerable to a lover translates into a lightness of being, our feet barely touching the ground we walk on! We no longer masquerade or hold back our total love in case our significant other might leave us, reject us for who we are; instead we experience a more complete love. Many of us are afraid to truly moan in ecstasy during the sexual experience. It is not merely that we are inhibited or repressed, but that we are afraid to make ourselves vulnerable. We wonder if we reveal our innermost joy, our significant other could break our hearts. Therefore we don't allow ourselves to get to that point. Instead we hold something back. It appears that sometimes we prepare for divorce the moment that we marry.

If we feel that we are special and unique beings, why fear the end of a relationship? When a partnership no longer works, we can move on in search of one that will be truly reciprocal. Because we have self-confidence, we believe that we will find someone else. Just like the job interview that didn't work out, another surely will. A better match will be made. We make ourselves vulnerable all over again as we become more experienced at it. Above all, when we have self-esteem, *we can find our true soul mate who resides within the self, not in another person.*

Vulnerability means being real in the relationship with the self. Let your feelings flow. You will feel more alive and experience more energy than you ever have before. If you are a strong, intelligent woman, look for a strong, intelligent man to mirror who you are and the same goes for a man. Do not suppress your personality because you worry that you will overwhelm a lover with your power. Make yourself truly vulnerable by expressing your strength and intellect. Be fabulous and live your truth! Only then will you attract the "right" person.

MIND/BODY PRESCRIPTIONS:

AID THE FLOW OF SELF-EXPRESSION

- ♦ Listen to your inner voice more. Even if you can barely hear your inner voice, keep listening as it will grow louder and more consistent with use.
- ♦ Don't judge your feelings. Acknowledge them.
- ♦ Look in the mirror and say, "I respect myself and am worthy of being loved." When you hold yourself in high esteem, others will too. Also, you will not be afraid to share your thoughts and feelings.
- ♦ After you have done your internal work, be the first one to express your feelings to a potential lover. Even if you are rejected, you will feel relieved, for you have released yourself from the prison walls of ambiguity, ready to embark on a new journey to your next happiness.
- ♦ If you are not rejected, but embraced instead, remember to be the first one to apologize when you have your first fight, especially when you believe you are right.
- ♦ When things have really worked out, allow your partner to create a night of passion for you—keep your eyes closed.
- ♦ Stand naked in front of your lover and let him or her stare at you for an indefinite amount of time.
- ♦ Fall back or forward into a trusted friend's arms.

MEDITATION:

Sit with dignity in a chair that makes you feel safe and comfortable with your palms facing up. Close your eyes and relax your breath. Inhale and exhale. Bring your attention to your heartbeat. Hear and see your heart beating. Allow your heart to expand with every breath. Feel it grow bigger and bigger until you feel as though you are all heart. In the center of your chest is a golden lock. Visualize the key in your hand. Now turn the key and unlock your heart. Breathe rhythmically. See a gold radiant light when your heart is open. Notice how the light forms a circle of your energy. Take a moment to read the name that floats in this radiant circle. Can you make it out? Does it surprise you? Hold your energy in your hand as you study and admire its powerful light. Take the time to fully experience your inner light. Then return your energy to your heart and leave it open. When you feel ready, return to your natural body. Let your heart return to its normal size and place of origin, but do not lock it. Open your eyes. Make a point of confessing your heartfelt feelings to the person whose name was locked in your heart. Was that person you?

EXERCISES TO BE VULNERABLE:

OBJECTIVE: TO STRENGTHEN THE BODY AS THE INTERNAL WALLS COME DOWN

Unilateral training as opposed to bilateral training concentrates an exercise to make the weak side stronger. This means that one arm, or one leg does the movement separately to make sure the other side is not compensating for that movement.

LEG PRESS
In the leg press add no weight except for the machine's resistance. Slowly press up from the heel of the left leg lowering to the chest in a deliberate fashion. Do not lock out the knee or let your hips curl up off the seat. After 8 repetitions, switch legs. Do 3 sets of 8. Advance to 25 per leg and add weights in gradual increments.

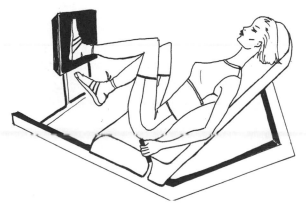

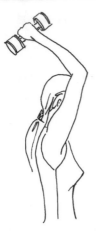

UNILATERAL TRICEPS PRESS

Grasp a dumbbell in your right hand (palm up) and raise it above your head, locking the elbow. Slowly lower the dumbbell behind your head until you feel a stretch in the triceps. Pause, then press the weight up above your head. Don't let the elbow flare out to the side. Keep it close to your head and pointed straight up. Do 8 repetitions. Switch to the left. Do 3 sets of 8. When that gets easy, increase the weight and do 3 sets of 12 repetitions on each side

UNILATERAL BICEPS CURL

Hold a dumbbell in your right hand. Extend your arm to full hang and then contract from the biceps muscle. The wrist comes along for the ride. Do 8 repetitions. Switch to the left. Do 3 sets of 8. When that gets easy, increase the weight and do 3 sets of 12 on each side.

UNILATERAL FRONT RAISE

Hold a dumbbell in your right hand in an overhand grip and extend out in front, level with your shoulder. Slowly lower all the way down and then slowly and deliberately lift up again. Do 8 repetitions. Switch to the left. Do 3 sets of 12. When that becomes easy, use a heavier weight and aim for 3 sets of 8.

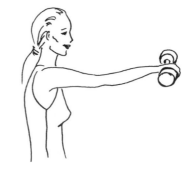

TRAINING TO TRUST IN A VULNERABLE SITUATION:

BENCH PRESS

The bench press provides a workout that recruits shoulders and triceps in addition to the pectorals because you must balance the bar--in contrast to the smith machine which balances for you and has a safety catch. If you lift at the bench press, a spot is recommended to assist you in this vulnerable position. Lie supine on the bench, knees bent, feet on the floor. Grip a 10-20 lb bar with hands shoulder width apart. Lower the bar to your chest then extend the bar straight up. Do not lock your elbows. Increase the weight progressively, 5 lbs at a time. Try a set of 8-10 repetitions. Work your way to 3 sets of 12 repetitions.

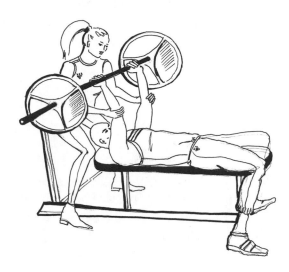

CIRCLE OF FRIENDS (*Not shown*)

Stand in a circle with friends, or people you trust. One at a time someone falls forward, right or left to be caught by another. A follow-up to this exercise is a meditation focusing on the person you chose to catch you and why?

CHAPTER 24

TRAINING TO BE INTIMATE

Folding clothes
I think of folding you
Into my life
Elisavietta Ritchie

O nce we have practiced being romantic which means living creatively and more spontaneously, we will create greater passion in our lives. Passion does not imply only sexual passion, but also translates into a passion for life. The intensity improves with practice. We can train ourselves to live more passionately by using our five senses and noting our feelings. Then we begin to speak openly about how we feel. We grow intimate with ourselves, ready to truthfully and continuously explore: Who am I and what do I want at this moment? We reveal our spark. Once we open up our hearts to a lover, we are ready to be intimate with another to give and receive: to speak in a beautiful language with a significant other that no one else can overhear or understand.

"YOU ARE THE MOST IMPORTANT PERSON IN MY LIFE. BUT THERE IS SOMETHING I HAVE TO TELL YOU. I DON'T KNOW HOW TO SKI."

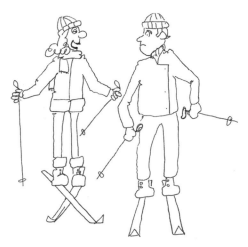

Intimacy is the highest form of truth between two people in a relationship. It is a complete comfort level where each member of the relationship is natural, communicating personal needs and desires. There are no pretense and false flattery. One can cry openly in a relationship. A lover can be silent and still understood.

Intimacy leads to commitment as two people feel secure in their love. Often communication takes place with a knowing glance. A concrete example of intimacy is sleeping in a lover's arms or in the spoon position after a sexual experience. This physical connection manifests the spiritual one. The special intimacy between a man and a woman combines the yin-yang of creation, the male-female energy of the life force or the union of opposites.

Intimacy between a couple flourishes because no one else on earth can duplicate their specific personal support system. What works for one specific couple, may not work for any other couple. For example, one couple thrives on compliments and an overt expression of sentimentality, while another thrives on a playfully competitive tug of war. However, in both cases there is an absence of guilt, nagging and submissiveness. Each half grows independently in career and personal development, contributing to the well being of the pair. In other words, the "couple" has distinguishable parts.

Intimacy is expressed and maintained in the small rituals couples create as a unit. For some it is sharing a drink before dinner, or taking a walk together after dinner. For others it is having breakfast together in the morning no matter how early one partner has to rise for work. For those who lead hectic lives there are weekly rituals like reading the Sunday paper in bed together, or going out to dinner as a couple one night a week.

Once intimacy has been achieved in a relationship, romance flows easily. Love is not a business deal that needs negotiation like if "I bring her flowers, take her out to dinner, she'll sleep with me tonight!" "If he buys me that pearl necklace, I'll give him a night to remember!" What matters is not the "material things" in the relationship, but rather time and attentiveness, the subtle statements: a knowing look, a whisper in the ear, an easy smile or a touch of the hand. While intimacy is born of romance, intimacy is its guardian, ensuring that the deep romance in a relationship never dies.

MIND/BODY PRESCRIPTIONS:

- ♦ Stand face to face with your lover about six inches apart. Stare into each other's eyes for five minutes without speaking. Do not move. You are permitted to cry. Remember: *two loving souls kiss through the eyes.*
- ♦ Read a love poem together.
- ♦ Write love letters to each other, or buy cards that express your feelings.
- ♦ Plan a weekend retreat with your lover in a serene setting. Hike together on nature trails and speak with your other senses. Do not talk. Take moments to notice the details about the other person. Listen to what is *not* being said.
- ♦ Plan a sexual interlude where you spend at least one hour of just touching and appreciating each other's bodies before having any sexual contact.

MEDITATION:

Sit comfortably with your palms facing up. Close your eyes. Inhale and exhale. Relax your breath. Imagine doing a laundry, a mixed wash of your "personals" and your significant other's. See your laundry whirl around with centrifugal force. Hear the change, hairpins, single lost earring, and matchbox hidden in a pants pocket clang in the machine. With your eyes still closed, look up to your eyebrows. Begin to feel as though you are floating with this experience. Observe how you remove the clean clothes from the machine and hang them individually on an outdoor clothesline. It is a balmy spring day, clear sky and country fresh. See the boxers, panties, shirts, skirts, pants, sheets and pillowcases swaying in the wind, billowing out. How do you feel when you watch a lifetime of laundry hanging outside? When the clothes are dry and ready, take them down from the line, sort and fold them. Be with your feelings as you fold your significant other's laundry. Sort out your feelings as you continue to sort out the laundry. Inhale the fresh scent of your lover's tee shirt. Exhale the stale pockets of resentment. Sense the essence of a life. Throw out any laundry you no longer need that has outgrown its use. Enfold to your heart the clothes that have special meaning for you because of their history. Smooth out the laundry and contemplate. Return to your body when you are ready. Open your eyes. Your laundry has been aired out and so have your feelings. Share this clarity with someone you love. Maybe you could even do your laundry together.

EXERCISES TO BE INTIMATE:

OBJECTIVE: TO ACHIEVE SYNCHRONY WITH ANOTHER

Asking for help, whether that person serves as a safety net, or whether that person actually assists in an exercise, one creates intimacy because energy and strength flow from one body to the other, almost undetectably. Sometimes that connection grows strong and one no longer has to ask for assistance because it is tacitly understood.

ASSISTED TRAINING

Assisted training helps you get beyond the sticking point. For example, if you are doing triceps presses and can no longer keep proper form as your muscles begin to fatigue, a partner can

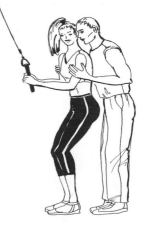

assist you to do a few more repetitions to recruit more muscle fibers. Resistance is reduced in accord with the muscle's contraction capacity as a partner helps you perform 2 or 3 post failure repetitions. Going beyond this capacity intensifies the training stimulus to increase muscle fiber development. When doing a triceps press, stand with your feet together and knees slightly bent. Using a high cable pulley, grasp a rope or bar with an overhand grip and tuck your elbows into your sides where they should remain throughout the movement. Press the bar down, (weight according to ability which you can increase over the weeks to come) while squeezing the triceps; then bring it back to upper chest level. Keep your wrists straight and do not rush. Try to do 3 sets of 10-12. In assisted training try to do 3 more beyond the burn.

TRICEPS PRESS AND CORE BALANCE

A triceps press on a stability ball recruits core balance. Holding a dumbbell in each hand in an overhand grip, weight determined by ability as you gradually go heavier, lie back on the stability ball to achieve support. Extend your arms overhead so that the weights are directly over your eyes. Keep your elbows in tight and your upper arms stationery. Holding your upper arms in a fixed position, slowly lower the weights until they almost touch your forehead. Pause briefly, then press back up slowly. At the finish, lock your elbows out. Try to do 3 sets of 10-12 gradually increasing to a heavier weight for 5-8 repetitions. When you feel that you can do no more, have a partner assist you by holding your arms stationary and try to do 3 more.

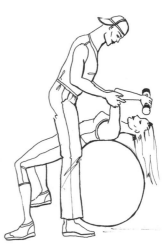

INTIMACY EXERCISE *(Not Shown)*

Sit cross-legged facing your partner with eyes closed. One partner has his palms facing up while the other has palms facing down. Both are focused on breathing: inhaling to the count of 4 and exhaling to the count of 6. You want to let go more than you take in. Work up to a count of 20 breaths. Begin to sense the energy from your partner, first from his hands and then his body. Allow your breaths to become in sync with one another. Feel the flow of energy as it leaves the body and enters you. Now repeat this exercise facing your partner with open eyes.

CHAPTER 25

TRAINING FOR THE BEDROOM

If ever two were one, then surely we
Anne Bradstreet

In order to feel sensual, energetic and creative in the bedroom, you have to train both your mind and body, preparing mentally and physically. Take a hot relaxing bath with aromatic salts. Dress in a costume to play the leading role in your fantasy. If you are not in the mood for a planned evening, then get in the mood by reading or viewing something sexually stimulating. It is as simple as that. If your partner no longer excites you, perhaps you need to excite yourself with a new outfit, music, fragrance or candles. Also, overall body conditioning enhances performance. Great sex is athletic because partners will go to great lengths to twist their bodies in a variety of positions and locations to make love. Excitement is generated by the strength and flexibility of each partner.

Stage the scene; direct it first through visualization and then implement indoors with candles, satin sheets, feathers, flowers and massage oils or outdoors with a picnic basket on a moonlit beach or in a lush garden. Nature refreshes the old routine. We should never consider love-making a duty, or a manipulative device for exacting what we really want. Sometimes we disassociate, or tune out, numbing ourselves from a joyous experience; for example, a woman will just let him "do it" to her while she composes her shopping list in her head, or a man watches the game on TV as he does it, wondering if the woman with him is asleep or awake.

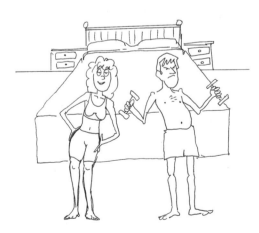

Be in the moment. Good sex obliterates all other concerns. Good sex reminds us that we are throbbing with life and loving energy. *An added benefit*: sex is youth enhancing; most notably it rejuvenates the skin.

A healthy diet helps promote quality lovemaking. Men need to avoid high cholesterol foods. Aside from being heart smart, this will prevent hardening of the arteries which decreases penile blood flow, one of the causes of impotence. Other factors that reduce potency are smoking and alcohol.

On the other hand women who starve themselves to look good, ironically, weaken themselves physically and alter their hormone levels. They become "starved for affection," with a dramatically decreased libido.

Exercise, specifically strength training, raises testosterone levels for both men and women, stimulating the libido. That is why training together provides good foreplay. Also, training will sculpt the body, firm it up, making it more attractive both to yourself and your partner. And if you feel more attractive, then your performance is far less inhibited in the bedroom.

The other day I was reading an article in a popular woman's magazine on how to camouflage unattractive body parts while making love. First and foremost, lingerie goes a long way towards hiding indiscretions. Then various positions were suggested to emphasize the body parts that look best while hiding the offending culprits. And once the man is actively involved, everything starts to look better to him, anyway; thus there is no need for anxiety in the first place. Interestingly enough, exercise, lifting weights and diet were not suggested in the article to improve appearance, stamina and pleasure. However, a compromise between the two approaches can be reached. While overall fitness and a healthy lifestyle are indispensable, lingerie and flattering positions can be useful in the interim or as a helpful prop in the bedroom to make you feel more attractive. Don't think of a relationship as a fifty-fifty partnership. Instead conceptualize it as one hundred-hundred. Sometimes you have to work overtime!

MIND/BODY PRESCRIPTIONS:

- ◆   Dance to release the sensual you and wear a costume.
- ◆   Relax your mind and body by soaking in a hot bath using candles and aromatherapy. Perhaps a glass of wine might help.
- ◆   Prepare favorite finger foods.
- ◆   Play music that has special meaning for both of you.
- ◆   Involve the five senses.

MEDITATION:

Visualize alone or preferably together. Close your eyes and lie down on your bed. Begin your breathing practice, letting your breath come and go. Sense the rising and falling of your chest and let your heart expand to the body of life. Loosen the ties that bind you to duty and daily concerns, allowing yourself to let go and float into a starlit universe. Continue to let all your cares melt away as you feel the tranquility of your center. Be one with your heart rhythm. Take a moment to experience this dreamy state. You are connected to the original source of love. Return to your heart energy. Know that it is the source of all inspiration. Your essence has been infused with love and serenity. Love flows in the rivers and streams of your body. Allow the gentle waters to find the path of least resistance. Smile to loosen the facial muscles that connect you to wholeness and love. Delight in the here and now and embrace the one who is close by. You can open your eyes if you like or keep them closed. Reach out…

EXERCISES FOR THE BEDROOM: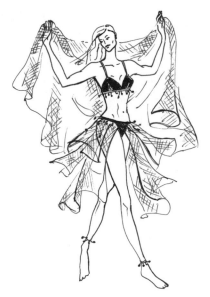

OBJECTIVE: TO SET THE STAGE FOR PHYSICAL PLEASURE

BELLY DANCING

Earthy movements will help you get in touch with your sexuality. Belly dancing shakes down inhibitions to release core female energy. A great workout for abdominals, quadriceps and rhomboids, the dance is done with knees bent, known as the motorcycle position, in order to freely rotate the hips. While ballet movements are angular and elongated, disciplined and carefully choreographed, belly dancing is circular and im-promptu, delighting in the roundness of the female form. Originating in the Middle East where women were cloaked and considered a father's, then a hus-band's possession, belly dancing enabled a woman to control her own space to express her sensuality. Most of the time women danced with and for other women to teach sensuality and subtle female expression. Belly dancing has existed for over 5,000 years, so there must be something to it! And when you dance for your significant other, you might not get to finish the dance… Similarly, Afro-Caribbean rhythms help release the female goddess within. Fertility residing in the powerful pelvic region is expressed in earthy move-ments that embrace sexuality. And if you seek a partner, Latin dancing provides a graceful and sensual release for two, rotating hips and arms in synchrony. Anyway, getting your partner involved in the dance is what the bedroom is all about.

NO BUTTS ABOUT IT!

While doing a gluteal workout off a stability ball, you tighten glutes, hamstrings and strengthen the pelvic region. Lie down on your back and position your heels on a stability ball. Get your balance. Tighten your abdominals as you lift up off the floor keeping your shoulders down and pull the stability ball towards you with your feet. Then push the ball back out. The heels are the driving force. Make sure you tighten your gluteals. Do as many as you can. Aim for 3 sets of 12 repetitions.

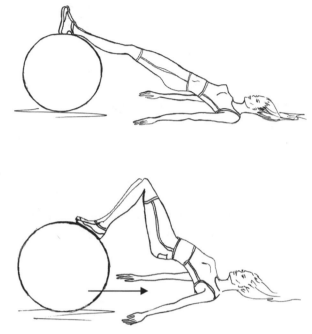

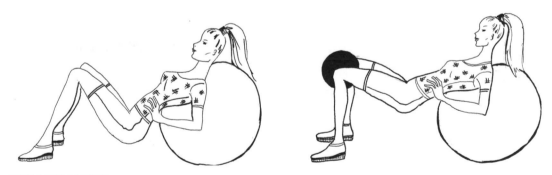

PELVIC LIFTS

Support your back on a stability ball as your legs are planted firmly on the floor shoulder width apart. Then lower your glutes almost to the floor, but do not touch, and as you tighten your glutes, push your inner thighs towards each other and lift your entire pelvic region up, like a bridge. Commonly this exercise is done on the floor without a ball. However, the stability ball enables you to begin from a higher position and go down low and then lift up for a greater range of motion. To increase intensity further, position a light ball between your thighs and squeeze the ball together as you do your pelvic tilts to work your inner thighs even harder. Aim for 3 sets of 12 repetitions.

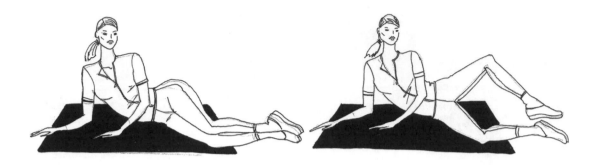

THE CLAM

To strengthen your inner and outer thighs lie down on your side tilting your pelvis and knees forward, one leg on top of the other. Then open your legs to form a diamond and bring your knees together, almost touching, slowly and methodically. Visualize moving against a resistance. Lift up and repeat. Open and close. Aim for 3 sets of 15 repetitions on each side.

TARGETS INNER THIGH

Support yourself on your elbow as you position yourself on your side. Extend both legs and bring your lower leg up using the adductor (inner leg) muscles to meet your raised upper leg (which is no higher than the hip and is stabilized in an isometric hold, providing a work-out for the outer thigh too). Then lower your leg back almost to the floor, slowly and controlled, but do not touch the floor. Aim for 3 sets of 15 repetitions on each side.

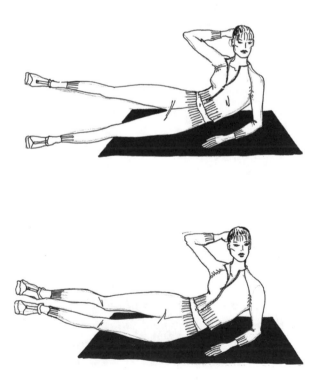

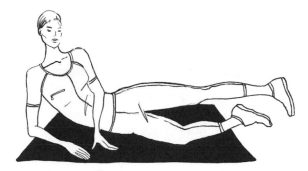

TARGETS BUTT AND OUTER THIGH

For that long lean look, lie down on your side and support yourself on your forearm. Extend your upper leg and point your foot down. Your lower leg is bent at the knee. Tighten your glute and leg as you lift your heel back on a diagonal, a couple of inches behind you. Note: this is a short, intense move. Do it slowly and rhythmically. Aim for 3 sets of 15 repetitions on each side.

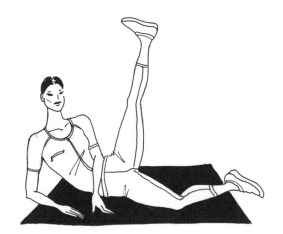

TARGETS OUTER THIGH AND BUTT

Lie down on your side and support yourself on your forearm. Bend the lower leg at the knee. Raise the upper leg straight up and extend directly in front of you- up and over- almost touching the floor. Aim for 3 sets of 15 repetitions on each side. Move slowly and controlled.

GET PHYSICAL!

Both men and women should do chest press exercises and push-ups: Men to increase strength, stamina and endurance; women to strengthen pectoral muscles to support the posture and carriage of the upper body which create the appearance of lifting up the breasts. A general cardio conditioning is necessary to ensure good performance (please see chapter 3, ***Training to Love Yourself***).

CHAPTER 26

TRAINING FOR TRAUMA

No Blow! No Blow!
They only ask the thing I turn
Inside the black ball of my mind,
The one white thought
Ann Stanford

No matter how cautious we are, no matter how in control we think we are, even if we have built a fortress and a moat, a traumatic experience can invade our psyche and steal our spirit. A violent act inflicts a blow to our self-esteem as we are rendered physically powerless, unable to prevent, or stop the assault. When we receive medical treatment, we are dependent on others for our physical care and restoration.

This chapter was inspired by Marla Hanson whose face was slashed by an attacker seeking to viciously mar her beauty and her modeling career simultaneously. Recently, when I saw Marla with her young daughter at a taping of a TV show in New York, she looked beautiful inside and out. She had reclaimed her spirit. She described how taking care of her daughter, nurturing a child, helped her find her way out of the darkness.

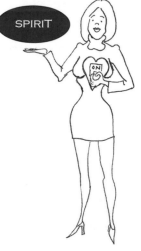

SPIRIT

When we experience trauma, we become the *victim*. Sometimes we see the face of our attacker. Peering into malevolent eyes of callous cruelty, we feel the assault more intensely, as it infiltrates our spirit. Other times even if our attacker is faceless such as if we are hit by a car and left to die, we might subconsciously feel that we are not worthy of being saved. Similarly, if we are beaten by a spouse, we might feel on some level that perhaps we deserved or triggered the violence. Then at night in our dreams the scene realistically or symbolically repeats. We begin to play a new role in life: the victim. People come to know us as the victim. As the walking wounded, we give ourselves permission to lick our wounds. We are now entitled to be legitimately bitter, easily angered, sleepy and unemployed. Our nearest and dearest have to tiptoe around us. The trauma that slashed, penetrated and crumbled our bodies has now settled into our soul driving away happiness, love, appreciation, forgiveness and compassion. The space is replaced by anger both overt and covert. While the body might heal on the outside, trauma has already changed the neurological patterns of our brains, perhaps responsible for some sort of disorientation occurring later in life, similar to the long term incubation of Mad Cow Disease. We could call it, "Spiritually-Angry Disease." The assault like being scalded by boiling water goes deeper and deeper under each of layer of skin, refusing to stop at the most superficial layer.

Many of the spiritual healers of our time shout, "Take back your spirit! Return it to the present, for it is trapped in the past outrage, in man's inhumanity to man." What is really being said, stripped of metaphor, is that one has to reclaim joy, delight in life by losing painful past history to live in the moment. Some victims do a good job of blocking out or disassociating from their traumatic experience; they suppress and suppress until, *the situation* is safely buried. However, because it is hidden, the pain burrows deeper, secretly doing its dirty work in the soul. Therefore if we don't know we have a problem, or disease, it can grow inward, unrestrained because we are not treating it. Conventional therapy helps a person overtly face his emotions to deal with them. Spiritual healers do the same metaphysically by inspiring the wounded to participate in his healing, facilitating extraction of the pain, which is accomplished through energy and touch. Some of us do it on our own, intuitively.

Recently, a forty-five year old woman in my belly dancing class related that she had awakened after a year-long coma, a result of being run over by a speeding car driven by a teenager. Miraculously, she recovered, yet had to relearn how to talk, walk, and remember. At first awkward and out of breath during class, over time her movements grew deliberate and graceful. Currently, she takes two workout classes a day and volunteers at the local library to boost her mental skills. The other day I asked her how she recalled her spirit. "At first I was so overwhelmed by the tragedy, I kept saying, 'why me? After all I am a religious woman and I do the right thing, why me, Lord? Then I heard my son say to me as he leaned over my bed, 'just get better, ma, just get better.' I realized that's what I had to do. I let go of my anger. I didn't hate the boy who ran me over anymore. It was at that moment that my son had recalled me to life. I was determined to get my life back." She smiled warmly. She didn't even have to share that she had reclaimed her spirit; I could see it in the way she danced. *It took Christ a long time to die, but a moment to rise.*

When we ask ourselves, "Why me?" or "What have I done to deserve this?" we are really saying that we have to justify the ways of God to man. The universe sends symbols and lessons to us that we often don't see or can't decode until later or never. We are too close to the big picture. Our salvation lies in forgiving the attacker to restore our power. We need to let go of the anger, the cry for justice. We release the energy drain of negativity to boost our energy bank. Hatred, anxiety, sadness and anger cost us energy. If we are too busy feeling negative emotions, we have no time to accomplish and enjoy. Before Christ was resurrected, he forgave his attackers for his murder. "Forgive them Father, for they know not what they do." Christ needed the energy to rise and he could not do it when he was weighted down by negativity, so he forgave his murderers. He needed to be lighter. Likewise those who suffer an attack must regain loving feelings in order to redeem their spirit. Forgiveness is in our self-interest: to release the negative feelings, which deplete us of our life force. Most of all, we must forgive ourselves for being victimized. Perhaps we didn't listen to our intuition and were at the wrong place at the wrong time. Perhaps we deplore our weakness at being unable to protect ourselves or stop the attack. We must forgive our sense of powerlessness. If we see the incident as part of the grand scheme of the universe and not as a punishment, we can accept our role in self-development. We might be motivated to embark on a new path, or even inspire the transgressor to change for the better.

Through our suffering we grow, expand and rise in ways we never imagined. When we overcome helplessness, we emerge empowered in new ways, stronger than we were originally. When we talk to others about our devastating experience, we teach and reinforce what we have learned. We create goodness. Now whatever we do is infused with greater understanding and appreciation. Through the contrast of evil we appreciate goodness. What we do with the dark spot in our lives is what matters, for it is only a spot in the ultimate scheme of things. By taking care of others who need our services we heal ourselves.

MIND/BODY PRESCRIPTIONS:

- ◆ Forgive your attacker. Say it; write it, as often as you need, until you mean it.
- ◆ Carry something heavy with you like a heavy pocket book, knapsack, or attaché case to symbolize your spiritual baggage. Then empty your baggage. Feel the lightness of being.
- ◆ Laugh or smile (if it is too difficult to laugh) no matter where you are every hour you are awake.
- ◆ Do not sleep beyond nine hours a night.
- ◆ Eat regularly whether you are hungry or not. Stay away from refined processed foods and sugar.
- ◆ Exercise daily after your doctor explains the do's and don'ts.
- ◆ Meditate at least once a day.
- ◆ Take care of someone else, a child, the elderly, or a pet.
- ◆ Surround your apartment or house with live plants for which you are responsible.
- ◆ Make sure to let in the light. Keep the blinds up in the daytime.
- ◆ Watch no more than an hour or two of TV a day. Avoid escaping into fantasy.
- ◆ Leave your home daily to go to work, go to lunch, or simply to walk outdoors.

- Join a support group. Talk about your experience and share with others. Bring the pain out into the open and then express the positive side of how it has changed your consciousness. Listen to what others have to say.
- Light a candle in a dark room. See the beautiful glow of illumination.
- Everyday do something you enjoy.

MEDITATION: 🧘

Sit comfortably with palms facing down. Close your eyes and relax your breath. Begin your breathing practice. Visualize a bare cherry tree in a lush garden. All is flowering in pink, purple, orange, red and yellow, except for the cherry tree in the center. Take a moment to experience the garden with your senses. Inhale the scent of the flowers. Hear the hum and the sweet song of birds and insects. Lean down to pick and taste the berries ripening on the bushes. However, the bare tree mars the rest of the garden, which is alive and full of summer scent. You miss the abundant white flowers and the deliciously tart red cherries cascading from its branches. What has happened to them? Where have they gone? Take a moment to reflect… Bring your attention to the tree. You think of cutting the tree down, yet hesitate because it has been your old friend for all these years and perhaps it could fit. See if you can keep this dead tree in your beautiful garden, which looks like a landscape painting. Bring your attention to your breath. A new inspiration gives rise to creative awareness. You gain access to a deeper place and something unusual emerges. Act on it. Pick up a can of paint, a brush and paint the tree a strong, dark vibrant blue. New feelings come up for you when you look at the tree sculpture in your garden. Take a long look and see how different and creative your garden has become. Feel a new energy take root. Experience for a moment how your body builds strong roots to support your beautiful spirit. You are grounded in nature and by nature. Your blue spirit is sun kissed and little yellow birds sing in your branches. You are filled with life and a new angle of vision. You have transformed insight into action and have demonstrated your ability to come up with creative solutions. When you are ready, return to your body with renewed spirit. There has been a shift from the ordinary to creative splendor. And deep inside you knew it all along. Gradually open your eyes to a new, hopeful perspective. You have the natural ability to color your life.

EXERCISES FOR TRAUMA:

OBJECTIVE: TO HEAL AND BECOME WHOLE

When you are physically able to do the following exercises after healing from physical trauma and the doctor permits, or even insists that you exercise, these workouts will help reaffirm life.

- *Step up and down a bench with ankle weights to symbolize the heavy baggage you carry. Then remove the weights and walk freely to experience a new easy step.*
- *Do a series of squats to stay grounded. Then after each squat, leap in the air to see how you rise. For squats please see chapter 27, **Training in the Garden**.*
- *Do dead lifts, making sure to rise to your full height at the end of each repetition. Please see chapter 17, **Training to Yield**.*

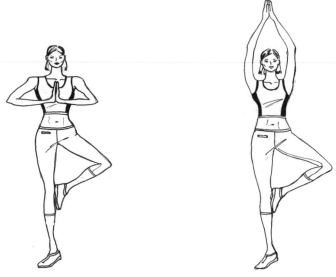

TREE OF LIFE
The Tree of Life posture develops concentration and balance. Although it is physically simple, it requires a clear inner focus. Stand up straight and balance on the right foot.

*The **beginner's level** is to bend the knee and position the foot against the opposite ankle.*

*The **intermediate level** (shown) is to position the foot against the opposite calf.*

*The most **advanced level** is to position the foot against the opposite inner thigh.*

***Note:** for all 3 positions the knee should be pointing outward. Next focus on a point straight ahead and bring both hands together in prayer position. Then keeping the palms together, slowly extend the arms above your head. Remember to breathe and try to hold this position for 5 complete breaths gradually increasing to 1 or 2 minutes. Repeat on the other side. This posture creates a special healing energy that lifts your spirit off the ground. If you think of the Kabalistic Tree of Life while you do this posture, you can feel your inner light ascending the branches of your own body.*

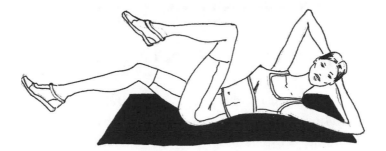

BICYCLES

Abdominals strengthen the core of the body from which all other movements derive power. Do the bicycle. Lightly support your head with your hands, press your back into the ground, lift off the right shoulder directing your right elbow towards your left knee and crunch; then reverse on the other side. As you pedal in the air, be sure to elongate the legs. Varying the "pedaling" angle, raising your legs higher or lowering them, targets a different abdominal area. If you wish to introduce a cardio burst, then you can pedal like the wind for a complete count of 10 and then slow it down to a natural rhythm as you pick up the pace once again for a count of 10. Try to do 3 sets of 25 methodical oblique crunches combined with 3 sets of 10 racing crunches. This exercise will help you move away from the painful past as you move towards new landscapes filled with joy, forgiveness and peace. As you bicycle, imagine life affirming thoughts to accelerate the healing process.

CHAPTER 27

TRAINING IN THE GARDEN

Tree at my window, window tree,
My sash is lowered when night comes on;
But let there never be curtain drawn
Between you and me
Robert Frost

It is fitting to conceive of gardening as one of the primal landscapes of physical fitness. After all, in parables of Western civilization mankind and womankind originated in the Garden of Eden. This idyllic setting was the first and most perfect home of Adam and Eve. All this makes sense. Gardens are natural sources of visual, tactile and olfactory delights. It is art that imitates nature, not vice versa. In many of the dominant religions stories and beliefs relate that man was created from earth and will return to earth. Therefore one can infer it is from the good earth that mankind receives his physical and spiritual sustenance.

In fact, we often speak of human "nature" when we analyze mankind. This suggests man as he once behaved in the Garden including his first disobedience and ensuing sense of shame when he was natural, stripped of pretense and a civilized veneer which obscures and confuses motives. And when the first couple was evicted from the perfect world of the Garden which involved little work on their part, one of their punishments was that Adam would have to work hard all his life, "By the sweat of his brow," to reap a harvest. Although not apparent at the time, God did Adam's muscles and bones a favor. Perhaps the first sin, the original one of disobedience, was part of a Divine physical fitness plan. Probably, that first edict, "Do not eat of the tree of knowledge" was meant to be broken, given human nature to be what it has been throughout the ages: bold, arrogant and then contrite. That is why so much of a gardener's work is performed on the knees, teaching us the humility we could never maintain for long.

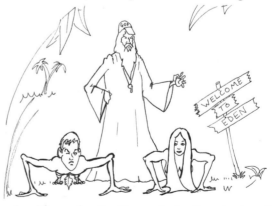

As Alexander Smith wrote in the nineteenth

century, "A man does not plant a tree for himself, he plants it for posterity," gardening helps keep us physically and spiritually fit, setting a wholesome example for the next generation.

Many current health articles report accumulating evidence that gardeners do not suffer from osteoporosis because of activities like digging and squatting to plant shrubs and trees, lifting heavy pots, bags of soil and fertilizer, or even pushing a lawn mower. Pruning, planting flowers and vegetables, especially cultivating hard-packed soil and pulling up weeds can elevate the pulse providing a bit of a cardio workout. Because gardening is a beloved hobby, gardeners tend to lose track of time, working hard for many hours, sustaining an activity level to be envied by avid gym members. *Note:* Because avid gardeners lose track of time, they do not age while gardening!

In addition, gardening is appropriate for all ages and genders. It produces attractive physical results in the gardener, creating a leaner body along with muscular arms and legs. Also, gardening is an exercise that creates a wholesome, serene environment of beauty and practicality as any flower, vegetable and fruit grower will testify. This imitation of the original Garden of Eden, a gardener's earthly delight, provides a graceful outlet for relieving stress and anxiety, lowering blood pressure and thus reducing the risk of heart attack and stroke.

In a world filled with politics, deception, prejudice, and man's inhumanity to man, isn't it wonderful to still have the natural gift of the garden in our spiritual legacy? We can have a little bit of heaven on earth.

MIND/BODY PRESCRIPTIONS:

A visit to your garden, your friend's or a formal botanical park will infuse your spirit and your body with serenity. A garden is a place where great changes occur; silently seeds push their way through the earth sprouting into leaves and flowers at their own pace without arrogance. Plant life does not seem to move in a garden, but there is constant movement and renewal. Seasonal changes parallel the seasons in our lives. Therefore we have much to learn by observing a garden. No winter lasts forever, for spring always makes its lively appearance, culminating in the treasure chest of summer. And summer needs to be cherished more than the other seasons, for it corresponds to the prime of life.

A garden during any season is a wonderful setting for meditation. Hard work and dreams combine to create a silent companion, teaching us to bring out the best in ourselves. The universe's handwriting is found in every garden; it is up to us to read the messages.

If you live in the city and don't have a garden and wish to exercise your green thumb, you can volunteer to work at a botanical garden or join community groups who transform overgrown city lots into secret gardens.

MEDITATION:

As you stroll along the pathways, find a spot that you are drawn to where you feel happiest or at peace. Notice what pleases you about your chosen space. Free yourself. Feel the positive rhythms of the garden. Is it the scent of a flower? The shady cool umbrella of a tree? Notice the sound of a waterfall cascading into an exotic lily pond. Sit down and really sense what nature offers freely. Inhale and exhale naturally. Observe the colors combining; hear the delicate rustling sounds. Allow your mind to expand and realize the timelessness of it all. Let nature permeate your senses. You have become one with nature.

EXERCISES FOR THE GARDEN:

OBJECTIVE: FOR EVERY GARDEN ACTIVITY A CORRESPONDING MUSCLE GROUP IS TRAINED

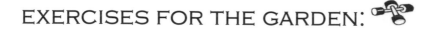

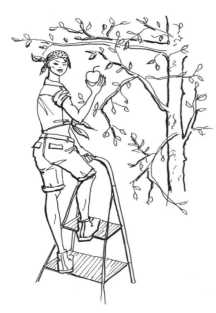

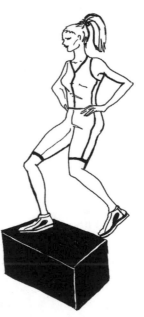

STEP UPS

Carefully step up and down an 8-12 inch high step. First do 8 repetitions on the right foot and then switch to the left. Try to do 3 sets progressing to 12 repetitions on each foot. Make sure your whole foot lands on the step. Hold abdominals in tightly and look straight at the horizon.

Eve climbs a step ladder to pick a ripe apple off her tree.

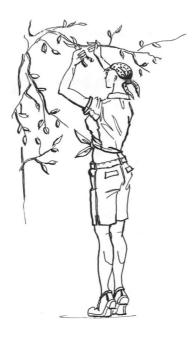

When you prune a tall shrub or low branches from a tree, often you stand on your toes.

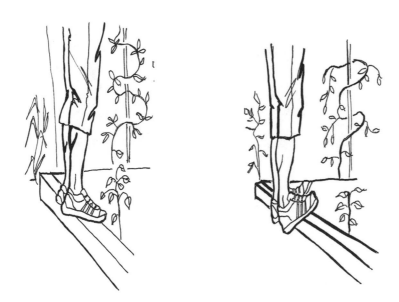

CALF RAISES
Stand on the last step with your heels hanging over the edge, holding on to a banister or a wall for stability. Then lift your heels as your weight shifts to the balls of your feet. Hold for 3 seconds. Lower your heels below the step for a full extension. Repeat for a set of 10-15 repetitions. Work your way up to 3 sets of 25 repetitions.

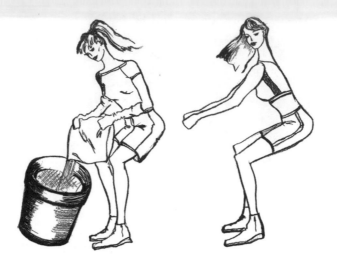

SQUATS

*Eve squats to unload soil into her planter. Then she demonstrates a full squat. Begin with feet shoulder width apart standing upright. Bend your knees tilting your pelvis back as though you were sitting down on a chair. In order to perform this exercise correctly, your heels need to be flat on the floor. **Hint**: Curl your toes up in your sneakers. Keep your shoulders back and chest out. **Important**: When you squat, make sure your knees do not extend over your toes. Return to a stand position with knees slightly bent. Begin with a set of 10-15 repetitions. Work your way up to 3 sets of 25 repetitions.*

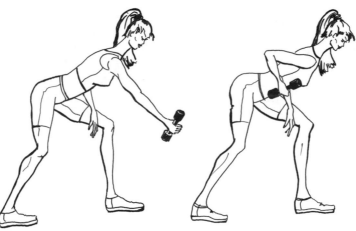

LOW ROWS

Eve demonstrates a one-arm low row, a move particularly useful in weeding. Stand in a lunge position where the left knee is bent, making sure not to extend the knee beyond the toes. The right leg extends with a slight bend in the knee. Contract the abdominals and make sure your back is flat. Shoulders are back and the right arm is fully extended in front of the body, with the left arm resting on the left knee. Pull your arm, so that your elbow goes beyond your back. Feel the middle of your back contract as you hold for 5 seconds. Release your arm to the starting position. The arm movement simulates a sawing motion. Repeat this exercise for 10-15 repetitions. Alternate to the other side. Build up to 3 sets of 20. Start with 3 lb weights and over time progress to 5, 8, and 10 lb weights.

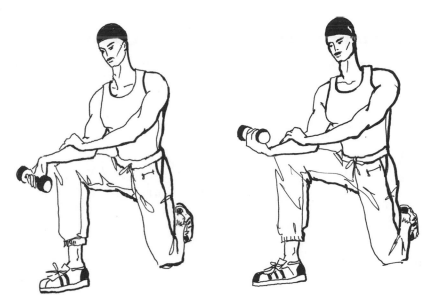

WRIST CURLS

The wrist curl strengthens the forearm for pruning. Kneel on one leg with your forearm supported by your bent knee, which is at a 90 degree angle. Your wrist hangs over the edge of the knee, dumbbell in hand. Flex your wrist; then curl up. Return to start position. **Note**: *This is a very small movement. Repeat this exercise for 1 set of 10 repetitions. Then alternate wrists. Work your way up to 3 sets of 15. Begin with a 3 lb dumbbell and for a more advanced move use 5 lbs.*

THE INTEGRATIVE POWER OF GARDENING

Gardening complements a comprehensive fitness program incorporating: walking, stretching and flexibility, finger dexterity, balance, strength, isometric holding positions, core stability and focus. These components frequently change depending on land, weather conditions and seasonal demands. Contraction, expansion, elongation and rest, all necessary building blocks of a sound body, parallel the components of plant life in a garden from the seed level and up. Plants and bodies adapt to their environment, transforming light into creative energy. A tree growing in the shade will alter its straight path to angle itself towards the sun, even if it has to distort its trunk. So too, will our path twist and turn in search of enlightenment and well being.

CHAPTER 28

TRAINING FOR THE YEARS OF GOLD

To see a world in a grain of sand
And a heaven in a wild flower.
Hold infinity in the palm of your hand,
And eternity in an hour
William Blake

What does it mean to be a senior citizen? Does the title command more respect? Does a person achieve the rank of seniority in life's experiences? Is a person considered an elder statesman? Unfortunately, quite frequently, the contrary is true. While senior citizens are given discounts at movie theatres, museums and other entertainment sites, many are prematurely "asked" to retire from their lifetime professions, dismissed as senile, unable to understand "modern" ideas, and relegated to rocking chairs, the way many infants are placed in swings and cradles that rock them automatically to keep them quiet. When a senior trudges up the stairs, or slowly crosses the street as the light changes against him, we want to scream, "Move out of the way," as we push aside or whiz past.

A common phrase used with senior citizens is, "Oh, he or she is in her second childhood." Childhood implies

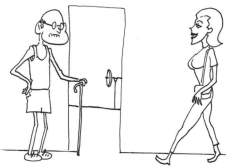

powerlessness and silliness. Children are told what to do by adults who either browbeat them to submission or actually beat them to behave according to their own prescribed mindset. In short, might makes right. To say that one is in his second childhood is to erode his authority.

SOMETIMES YOU NEED A LITTLE MOTIVATION

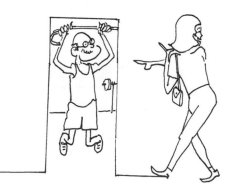

However, the inevitable weaknesses and diseases that remain inherent in the aging process create a keen awareness that the body is a repository for the soul. Therefore when caretakers bathe, diaper and dress the weakened body, the soul is not degraded, but instead is separating itself from the body to assume its true identity. While Eastern philosophy reveres the wisdom of old age, our throw-away society dismisses many of the keen perceptions of the elderly with, "They simply do not understand or remember what it feels like to be young." In fact, youth enhancing products are called anti-aging! That sounds insulting.

As we age, we come to realize that experience is a great teacher. George Bernard Shaw aptly assessed the situation: "Youth is wasted on the young." As people age, they grow less distracted by trivialities, less diffuse in their focus. Because time becomes a consideration, more than with young people who tend to believe that they are immortal, life grows more intense and sweeter.

A famous Zen parable presents an enlightened riddle depicting the aging process: a ferocious tiger was chasing a man, hungrily eyeing him as his next meal. The man ran until he arrived at a precipice where he had to make a choice: jump or be eaten. He took hold of an old deeply rooted vine and swung down, dangling over the edge. The man looked down to see where he might land. To his dismay another tiger waited below. The man trembled realizing his fate. Meanwhile two mice, one black and one white, were gnawing at the vine that suspended him in temporary safety from the two tigers. Suddenly the man noticed a luscious strawberry within his reach. Relaxing his grasp on the vine, he held on with one hand as he reached for the strawberry with the other. How delicious that strawberry tasted!

The point of this succinct parable is that as an older person clings to his deeply rooted vine, his earthly connection, he knows how to taste life, to live intensely and in the moment. Because he is more conscious about time passing, he appreciates a simple joy, which is too often overlooked. A senior citizen is more likely to have a fresh and appreciative outlook on life than a young person. Consider this: sunrise and sunset appear the same—it all depends which direction you are facing, east or west.

With medical science enabling us to live longer, more of us are becoming members of the golden years club, finding ourselves strong mentally and physically, eager to contribute to the community and to live life fully. When I celebrated my mother's seventy-fifth birthday, I asked her how she felt having lived three quarters of a century, which sounds much older than seventy-five. She cheerily commented, "I simply don't feel my age. When I look in the mirror, I am surprised to see the face of an old woman greet me because I still feel like a young girl." For most of her life my mother marched briskly everywhere she went, carrying packages before it became trendy to fitness walk with weights, keeping herself vibrant and peppy, as she managed a business.

What comes to mind about the journey of the senior citizen is a poem written by Alfred, Lord Tennyson passionately depicting an aging legendary Greek hero, Ulysses, who still longs to go on adventures and discover new worlds. He refuses to yield to old age, "How dull it is to pause, to make an end;" instead the aging king seeks renewal and reinvention: "To follow knowledge like a sinking star." In the following excerpt from this famous poem, the heart and soul of a spirited senior citizen is explored.

> *You and I are old;*
> *Old age hath yet his honor and his toil.*
> *Death closes all; but something ere the end,*
> *Some work of noble note, may yet be done,*
> *Not unbecoming men that strove with Gods.*
> *The lights begin to twinkle from the rocks;*
> *The long day wanes; the slow moon climbs; the deep*
> *Moans round with many voices. Come, my friends.*
> *'T is not too late to seek a newer world.*
> *Push off, and sitting well in order smite*
> *The sounding furrows; for my purpose holds*
> *To sail beyond the sunset, and the baths*
> *Of all the western stars, until I die.*
> *It may be that the gulfs will wash us down;*
> *It may be we shall touch the Happy Isles,*
> *And see the great Achilles, whom we knew.*
> *Tho' much is taken, much abides; and tho'*
> *We are not now that strength which in old days*
> *Moved earth and heaven, that which we are, we are,--*
> *One equal temper of heroic hearts,*
> *Made weak by time and fate, but strong in will*
> *To strive, to seek, to find, and not to yield.*

It is in the spirit of Ulysses that the exercises for senior citizens will be approached in this section. Sometimes old age is accompanied by a form of physical frailty. Many emotional up-heavals can potentially create an even greater spiritual frailty. Widows and widowers might experience an identity crisis that leaves the surviving partner feeling like half an equation. In addition, retirement might remove direction and obscure purpose intensifying the identity crisis. With no more children to raise, the death of a spouse, and no job to structure daily life, seniors seek to redefine and reaffirm their goals.

Exercise for the golden years should promote quality of life and independence: *movement that matters*. Exercise programs strive to increase basic functions such as dress, hygiene, diet and mobility. In addition, other exercise programs concentrate on more advanced functional demands: housework, food preparation, driving, shopping and mental acuity. Strength training is geared to build bone and muscle mass preventing osteoporosis. Stretching will increase flexibility and thus ward off arthritic stiffness and ligament injury. Aerobic fitness will help combat depression, as well as lower blood pressure to create a heart smart body. Even where there has been a previous heart attack or stroke, exercise after a physician's approval, can help ward off any further episodes. Widespread studies have shown that it is *never too late* to begin a fitness program. And even where there has been prior bone loss, seniors can still increase their bone density through weight training to prevent further debility from osteoporosis. In addition, mental acuity becomes a benefit as more oxygen suffuses the brain during physical exercise. As seniors perform new exercises, learning new patterns of movement, fresh neural pathways are created in the brain alert to new thoughts. "Live and learn."

Training the body and the mind become equally important in this age category. Workouts concentrate on enhancing function and mobility. Also, seniors want to enjoy life as active participants, not mere spectators. Above all, a positive attitude and a strong motivation during exercise to push through the iron gates of life will create a renewal of the life force, a youthful reflection on one's relationship to the ultimate scheme of things. How often do we hear about people in their eighties and nineties discovering love and romance, beginning a deep commitment to one another! Love is ageless! Self-realization is ageless!

In Kung Fu meditations a four-line poem succinctly clarifies the two opposing approaches one could carry into old age: Which would you choose?

> *In the light of the setting sun,*
> *Men either beat the pot and sing*
> *Or loudly bewail*
> *The approach of old age.*

We prepare ourselves on earth for the next journey to a new location; perhaps, each one of us has a personal theory to explain the riddle of existence.

It is strongly recommended that aside from a medical evaluation, a senior citizen beginning an exercise program should do so with a fitness professional, for at least the first few sessions. A professional will assess fitness level through an interview and observation. First hand observation proves to be invaluable, revealing problems and weaknesses often not admitted by the client. During the interview questions will be posed to the client: Why are you here? What do you want to do in your life, or what do you want to do again? A trainer will pay strict attention to form, as he works together with his client to prevent injury, increasing range of motion and fitness and promoting good health to achieve a mutually desirable program goal. A trainer will also teach the client to listen to his or her body. Workouts for the golden years should be *pain free* (no pain, no gain, does not apply here) and *consistent*.

Another option for a workout is to attend classes geared specifically for senior citizens, such as body sculpting or dance. Regularity and consistency are achieved through scheduled times and places, minimizing workout cancellations or excuses like, "Not today, I'm tired." The advantage of specialized classes at gyms or senior centers is group energy, which fuels the individual. "If others can do it, I can do it." Other benefits of attending classes are: getting out of the house, making new friends along with cultivating a regular social support group to have fun as endorphins rise.

MIND/BODY PRESCRIPTIONS:

REJUVENATING ACTIVITIES

- Find hobbies that you love to do. When you lose track of time, you don't age.
- Listen to different music; watch a different TV show.
- Intend to grow younger and live longer.
- Learn something new everyday; it can be as simple as a new vocabulary word.
- Practice conscious breathing to energize as well as soothe mind and body.
- Avoid toxic foods and drinks along with toxic relationships.
- Volunteer as a grandparent to a lonely, troubled child.
- Attend programs at senior centers to meet people and make new friends.
- Write your memoirs as a legacy to future generations. Questions and answers to be shared with younger members of your extended family:
  - Knowing what you know now, what would you have changed in your past?
  - What preparations would you have made for this stage of life?
  - What advice would you give someone forty years old?
  - Someone twenty years old?

MEDITATION:

Sit comfortably on a chair, close your eyes. Keep the palms of your hands open and facing up. Breathe consciously; inhale and exhale to relax your breaths. Continue to breathe to your own rhythm. Visualize a life-size mirror framed in jewels suspended in mid air. Approach the mirror and peer into it. What do you see? Do you see yourself according to your chronological age or your internal age? Allow this image to escort you on a journey to your past. Choose a memory like your honeymoon night, your child's first day of school, or your first job. Pass through the mirror and merge with your reflection. Take a few moments to reflect on who you once were and who you want to be now. Continue to inhale and exhale. Breathe mindfully. Be there suspended in time and place. Are you happy with what you see? Is there some aspect of yourself you wish to change? Allow this transformation to take shape to help you become the person you want to be. Are you happy with this vision? If not, let it assume another shape which causes you to smile at your new image. Become one. Slowly, begin to return to your surroundings. Come back to your body. Carry this new-found impression internally as you stride through the mirror. Awaken to joy and openness.

EXERCISES FOR THE YEARS OF GOLD:

OBJECTIVE: TO IMPROVE STABILITY, COORDINATION AND BALANCE

Workouts should be performed for a minimum of two days per week with forty-eight hours of rest between sessions. Thirty minutes is the optimum time for a session. An hour is the absolute maximum, performing at first eight to fifteen repetitions per set and then twelve to twenty repetitions that demand some exertion.

In the beginning for the first two months workouts should use light resistance to allow the muscles and ligaments to adapt. Proper breathing is emphasized. This sets the foundation for a lifetime commitment.

Moving on to the next level should involve first, increasing the number of repetitions and then increasing weight. Performing multi-joint exercises is preferred to performing single joint exercises. If possible, machines are preferred over free weights as they are less likely to cause injury and easier to manage than free weights. Special concerns in senior workouts: frozen shoulder, rotator cuff injury, biceps impingement and keeping the humerus below shoulder level when arms are raised.

Do 10 to 15 repetitions of each the following. For a more advanced workout use a heavier ball, heavier weights, or a trainer can add a safe and appropriate resistance.

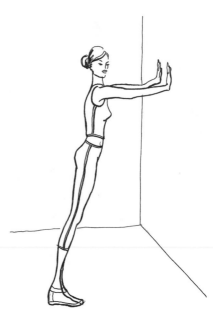

WALL PUSH-UPS FOR THE CHEST

*The traditional exercise is the seated chest press and the push-up. This home version is equally effective in improving the ability to push and carry packages while shopping or closing and opening doors: Place hands on the wall shoulder width apart and do push-ups standing up. Hand positions change up from narrow to wide. **Tip:** Keep shoulders down through movement.*

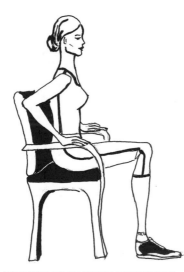

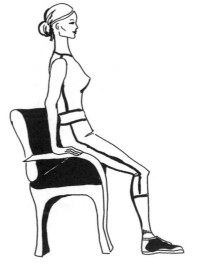

CHAIR PRESS UPS FOR TRICEPS

When seated, place hands outside of thighs on the arms of your chair and press the body up.

BICEPS CURLS *(Not Shown)*

*First do a curl with no weights and then with light weights gradually increasing resistance as you contract the biceps. The wrist (keep it straight and stable) comes along for the ride. For seated biceps curls please refer to chapter 1, **Training to be Conscious**.*

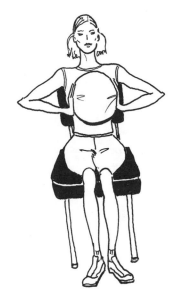

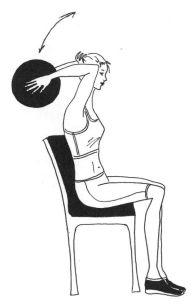

CHEST PRESS SQUEEZE

Hold a balloon or ball in front of you with hands about chest height. As you squeeze the ball, extend your elbows.

TRICEPS

Place a ball or balloon in hands positioned behind the head, lift and lower.

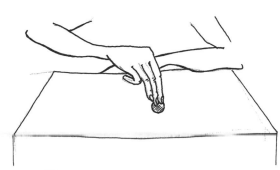

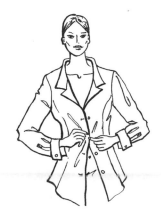

FINGER DEXTERITY

Turn a penny over and pick it up to help arthritic fingers stay nimble to button and unbutton a shirt.

OTHER EXERCISES FOR THE YEARS OF GOLD

- ◆ *To improve reaction time and hand-eye coordination*
  - ◆ *Throw a ball and catch it.*
  - ◆ *Play Simon Sez.*

- ◆ *To improve grip strength, finger coordination and help arthritic fingers*
  - ◆ *Open and close your hands.*
  - ◆ *Squeeze a tennis or Koosh ball.*
  - ◆ *Crumple a sheet of newspaper and squeeze it in your hand to promote finger dexterity.*

NOTE
Exercise intensity should correspond to the length of time you have been training. Crawl, walk and run. As you become more fit and stronger, progress to more challenging exercises.

CHAPTER 29

TRAINING TO TAKE YOUR OWN ADVICE

*Only when a man is safely ensconced
Under six feet of earth, with several
Tons of enlauding granite upon his
Chest, is he in a position to give advice
With any certainty, and then he is silent*
Edward Newton

Throughout the ages kings have appointed counselors, prophets and ministers to advise them; of course, let us not forget the role of magicians and Shakespearean "fools" in this entourage. Presidents carefully pick their cabinet members. We select our good friends to confide our trusted secrets and to hear their advice. Many of us enjoy playing the role of the "wise one," the teacher. We tend to feel empowered and respected. For example, we tell the *angry* friend to calm down and analyze the situation. We tell the *highly emotional in-love* friend to think before making a commitment. We tell the *steeped in-sorrow* friend to get over it. We can be hailed as experts at giving advice, especially if we give it freely and with enough conviction in our voices; no certification or apprenticeship is necessary. Yet, how often do we heed our own advice when we are upset, heartbroken or in love? Do we practice what we preach?

When my friend is fuming, the anger burning in fiery flames from the top of her head, I tell her to visualize and breathe deeply. I dissect the scenario and make her see that she is

WE MUST ALWAYS
BE PEACEFUL

SHUT UP!!

OHM...

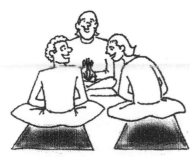
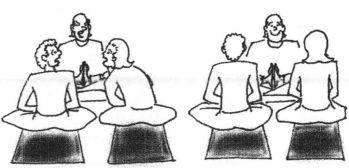

overreacting. However, when I am angry, I do not breathe deeply and visualize enchanted gardens, even though I am a gardener, or analyze the situation to realize that I overreacted. Instead, I scream, rip out weeds and tear a lot of paper napkins imaging various body organs of the person at whom my rage is directed.

My trainer loves to recite proverbs, particularly those that are Zen inspired, comprising the dualities of human existence. Some are quite poetic and hit the spot when he senses my specific personal upset. However, when he feels angry and dismayed and I return the favor with my own proverbial repertoire, which is quite literary I might add, I receive a gruff retort, "Now, *you're* quoting *me* proverbs!" I mumble under my breath, "Apparently, you do not practice what you preach!" I make sure not to tell him this critical piece of advice during our training session. As was discussed in *Training To Shut Up,* I have learned to keep my mouth shut and I heed my own advice in this instance as we are doing resistance training with him applying the resistance!

Apparently advisors need their own advisors to keep them in line and supervise them. We preach to people who mirror our own issues, consciously or subconsciously. We can give advice objectively regarding the issue that is presented, even though it might actually be our own problem which is conveniently housed in a friend. In helping *our friend* figure it out, we are really trying to help ourselves work it out.

By acting as an advisor we sharpen the tools we need to use in order to take care of ourselves. By teaching others, explaining the concepts to others, we learn them more thoroughly. When we tutor someone in a subject of our own expertise, we understand the subject better after we have taught it. If we do not heed our own advice, then the universe will send us new friends who need to hear the advice that we are meant to take. The cycle will continue and we will repeat our words until we hear them in our hearts and in our minds.

Therefore the next time you spout proverbs, directions for living and psychological tidbits, remember that the advice you are giving to your friend is the advice you need to internalize. And when you are most angry with your friend, perhaps you are most angry at what that friend is mirroring in you. And if you don't practice what you preach, then stop preaching! Myself included!

MIND/BODY PRESCRIPTIONS:

- ♦ When you are emotionally upset, substitute your friend's name in that personal scenario.
- ♦ Stand in front of a mirror and look at yourself as you pretend to advise a friend.
- ♦ Bless the person who has triggered your emotional response. Forgive his or her humanity and in so doing you will release yours.
- ♦ If you still find yourself advising a lot of people, reread *Training To Shut Up.*

MEDITATION:

Sit up with dignity, palms facing up; close your eyes and relax your breaths. Find yourself on a long winding road on a hazy day with the morning fog just starting to burn off. Notice your surroundings: the trees, the hard-packed earth beneath your feet, the wild flowers. Your journey becomes more determined. You sense that you are not alone-- as if your hand is being held. Down the road you see a distant figure. As you move forward on your path, you realize that you know this figure. Take a moment to reflect on your feelings to see if you can identify who this person is or what he or she represents. You smile with recognition: this familiar person is your spiritual guide and has a gift for you. It is beautifully wrapped and given with an open hand. You accept the gift. If you have any questions that need guidance, you can now ask them of your spiritual guide. Notice that the answer may not come in the form of a word at this time. It may come later in the form of a sight or a sound. The answer may even be housed in the gift. Thank your guide and continue on your way knowing that you have received Divine guidance. Open your present and see what is inside. Whatever comes to mind first is your gift. Don't judge; rather accept and feel the emotions that come up for you. Be with this experience for a few moments. When you are ready, return to your reality carrying this present with you. Trust your inner knowing because the guide you have thanked is a part of you. Open your eyes.

EXERCISES TO TAKE YOUR OWN ADVICE:

OBJECTIVE: TO OBSERVE AND PARTICIPATE AT THE SAME TIME

TRAINER AND CLIENT
ENERGIZE ONE ANOTHER
WORKING TOGETHER
IN AN EXERCISE BOUT
TELL - SHOW - DO

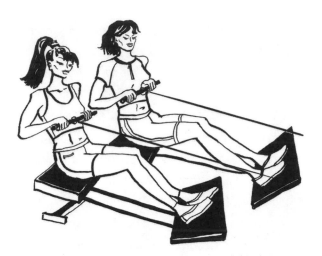

ROWING MACHINE

Trainer and client do the rowing machine: Keep your back straight, abdominals in, elbows back and chest out with every pull, squeezing the shoulder blades. Begin with 5 minutes and work your way up to 20. This is a good cardiovascular exercise for the upper body since most people do aerobic exercises for the lower body and neglect the upper body.

CHIN-UPS

Trainer and client do chin-ups. Grab the bar underhand (palms up) with hands shoulder width apart, body hanging from the bar. Knees are bent and your partner holds your feet for slight assistance during a sticking point. Pull up bending your elbows and lead with the chest to the bar. Tighten your abdominals to support your lower back. In the beginning you might want to rest your feet on your partner's thighs who will then give you a bigger boost from that position. Try to do as many as you can. When you adapt to this exercise, try to do 3 sets of 10.

SPRINTS (*not shown*)

Trainer and client sprint together to spur each other to compete and quicken the pace. Sprints (short running bursts) recruit fast twitch muscle fiber, triggering your body to lean out. Jogging is an aerobic workout which tends to lean out muscle mass as well as burn fat. However, sprinting is anaerobic and burns only fat. Alternate a 10 second sprint with 1 minute walking. As you build up your stamina, increase your time to 20 minutes, alternating sprinting and walking.

FAREWELL
TO THE READER

Writing a training for life book, presenting advice for the mind/body love knot, has triggered a personal exploration for the author, the fitness professional and the artist, "Physician heal thyself," so to speak. We have combined different cultural and life experiences, artistic inspirations, and creative training to help the reader learn how to turn on his inner light, illuminating the happiness that life presents. Each one of us has to face what we most need to learn about ourselves, leading to an understanding of the larger context of humanity.

Together author and reader confront individual demons, weaknesses, stressors, sorrows and triumphs. These pages form our mutual and binding journey. We perceive them to be a glowing light in a dark room. If you find even one chapter that changes or enhances your perception about a life situation, or provides you with a coping skill, then grasp it as a lit candle in your hand. As a myriad of individual candles, we can glow as a universal we instead of separate I's.

ABOUT
THE AUTHOR

Debbie Eisenstadt Mandel awakened with a jolt early one March morning two years ago with the inspiration to write this book. She conceptualized a book presenting a creative merger of fitness and spirituality as a comprehensive response to the question: "Debbie, why are you so happy? If I didn't know you so well, I would think you must be on something!" Paradoxically, yet in complete accord with metaphysics, Debbie has confronted the darkness to appreciate the light. She is a second generation holocaust survivor who is determined not to survive, but to really live. She believes that nowadays when we live longer, we need to learn to live more fully and with a sense of humor.

Debbie received her undergraduate and graduate degrees from Brooklyn College (Summa Cum Laude) and New York University respectively and was elected to the Phi Beta Kappa honor society. In addition to teaching English literature and writing on the high school and college levels, she has devoted years to studying and developing a panoramic and analogous view of Chinese herbal medicine, health and fitness, Western medicine, Zen philosophy, Kabalistic healing and literary patterns. This creative merger of archetypes, stories and science gives shape and depth to her theme: a journey toward recognizing and appreciating the essentials of happiness. By freeing the self from the past story, one can create the present story. Living in balance: physical, intellectual, emotional and spiritual, is the source of energy and joy.

Debbie is married, a mother of three children and a dog. She is an ardent gardener and landscaper. She exercises regularly, meditates and belly dances.

Debbie is a noted speaker and runs frequent workshops in the New York City area on various topics associated with de-stressing and cultivating an eye for joy, including: *Training to be Conscious, How to Fall Asleep and Stay Asleep, Boost Your Immune System, KIND (Kids In Need of De-stressing), How to Turn Stress into Strength, Fend Off Fatigue* and *Turn Back the Clock... Grow Younger.*

For additional information please visit busybeegroup.com. You can contact Debbie by fax at (516) 371-1398 or via e-mail debbie@busybeegroup.com.

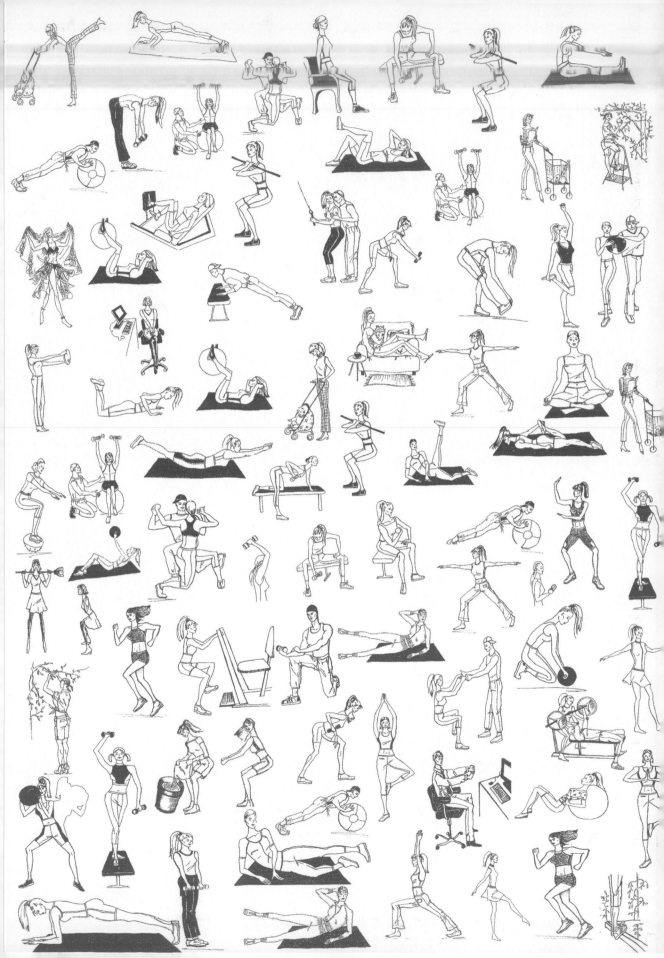